# Slide Interpretation for the MR

# Slide Interpretation for the MRCP

## Hugh J. Kennedy MD MRCP
Consultant Physician to
the Norwich Health
District, UK

## Timothy W. Evans BSc PhD MRCP
Senior Registrar, Brompton Hospital, London;
formerly Research Fellow, Academic Division
of Medicine, University of Sheffield, UK

## Andrew Suggett PhD MRCP
Senior Lecturer in Medicine,
University of Sheffield, UK

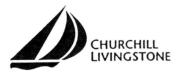

CHURCHILL
LIVINGSTONE

EDINBURGH LONDON MELBOURNE AND NEW YORK 1987

CHURCHILL LIVINGSTONE
Medical Division of Pearson Professional Ltd

Distributed in the United States of America by
Churchill Livingstone Inc., 650 Avenue of the
Americas, New York, N.Y. 10011, and by associated
companies, branches and representatives throughout
the world.

First published 1987
    Reprinted 1994
    Reprinted 1996

ISBN   0-443-03638-1

**British Library Cataloguing in Publication Data**

Kennedy, H.J.
    Slide interpretation for the MRCP.
    1. Symptomatology—Problems, exercises, etc.
    I. Title   II. Evans, Timothy W.
    III. Suggett, Andrew
    616'.0022'2    RC69

The
publisher's
policy is to use
**paper manufactured
from sustainable forests**

Produced by Longman Asia Ltd, Hong Kong
GC/03

# Preface

The examination for Membership of the Royal College of Physicians (MRCP) consists of two parts. In the first, knowledge is tested by multiple choice questions. In Part II, there are a written paper, viva and clinical cases. The written paper is divided into three sections which are: the analysis of case histories (the 'grey' cases), a section on the interpretation of data and a slide session. The candidate has to pass this 'written' paper before being allowed to progress to the clinical cases and viva. The exam is designed to select those candidates suitable for higher medical training. Its aim is to test observation, clinical competence and knowledge. Most failures result from inadequate preparation and poor technique. The slide interpretation section consists of 20 compulsory questions, each based on a slide. Two minutes are allowed for each, with a bell being rung after one-and-a-half minutes to give warning prior to the change of the picture. Up to a third may be X-rays, which are considered in a companion volume of this book: *X-ray Interpretation for MRCP* by Charles R.K. Hind. We give examples of the remainder in this volume, including clinical, ophthalmology, haematology and histopathology slides.

We have divided the 100 questions in this book into 5 papers with 20 photographs in each. Look at the picture and read the question carefully, as it may contain a helpful clue, then study the slide again. The main abnormality may be obvious but it is important to inspect the rest of the picture for other clues. For example, a full frontal picture of a patient with acromegaly may show the facial appearance with prognathism and large hands and feet but there may also be a lack of pubic hair suggesting hypopituitarism following therapy.

Answer each question or each part of the question precisely and accurately. Each has a preferred answer which will obtain maximum marks but sensible alternatives also gain marks. Do not either panic if you are unable to answer a question, or continue to try to answer one when the next slide is shown.

Allow 40 minutes for the 20 questions in each paper. It is important to write down your answers before consulting those accompanying each paper. The information given in the answers in a book of this size are inevitably brief. Therefore, it is often helpful to read more detailed texts about the subjects illustrated in the slides.

Norwich, London and Sheffield                    H.K.
1987                                             T.E.
                                                 A.S.

# Acknowledgements

We are deeply indebted to Dr M. Greaves, Dr A. Kennedy
and Mr J.F. Talbot for the use of their slides and for their
expert opinion and advice. We are most grateful for the
considerable time and effort that they gave so willingly to
help us. We should like to thank Professor S. Tomlinson, Dr
J.D. Ward and Dr J. Francis for their enthusiastic support
and for allowing us to use some of their excellent
photographs. Finally, we should also like to thank the
Departments of Medical Illustration at the John Radcliffe
Hospital, Oxford, and the Royal Hallamshire Hospital,
Sheffield, for their permission to reproduce illustrations
from their collections.

# Contents

# Paper 1

# Question 1.1

This child was brought to casualty: what investigation would you do?

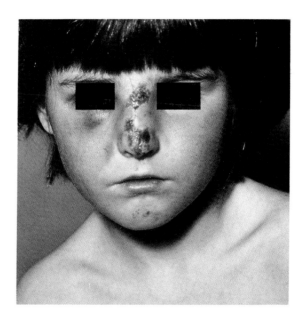

## Answer to question 1.1

A skeletal survey.

This is a case of non-accidental injury. Battered babies account for about 100 deaths in the U.K. each year. It is not a typical case because bruising and lacerations to the face are unusual. Other features include:

(a) Bony injuries, especially to the ribs and long bones. Subperiosteal haematomas, displaced epiphyses and avulsion injuries are also common.
(b) Bruises may be multiple and of different ages.
(c) Head injury: skull fracture and subdural haematoma may occur together or separately. Retinal and subhyaloid haemorrhages are a common accompaniment.
(d) Burns, either from cigarettes or holding the child close to a fire.

Suspicious points in the history include inexplicable delay in seeking medical help and incompatibility between the history and the extent of the childs injuries. It should be remembered that child abuse may involve psychological and sexual abuse as well as physical injury.

# Question 1.2

How would you confirm the diagnosis?

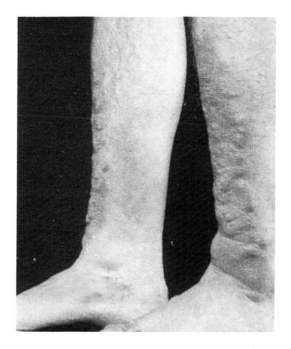

## Answer to question 1.2

Serum $T_3$ and $T_4$.

Pretibial myxoedema derives its name from the deposition of mucopolysaccharides in the subcutaneous tissue of the legs. They begin as small plaques and coalesce to give a peau d'orange reddish pink colour. It has to be differentiated from hypostatic and lymphoedema. It is most commonly associated with hyperthyroid eye signs and rarely clubbing. Treatment is of the thyrotoxicosis but the deposits may remain even when the patient is euthyroid. Intralesional injections of steroids have been tried.

# Question 1.3

This is a microscopy specimen of stool from a patient with loose motions. What is the diagnosis?

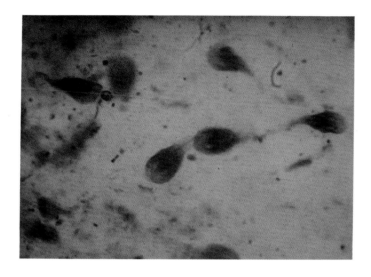

## Answer to question 1.3

Giardiasis.

*Giardia lamblia* is a flagellate parasite with a worldwide distribution especially in the tropics but is endemic in Eastern Europe and the USSR. The parasite is recognisable by its pear shape (up to 20 μm long by 15 μm wide) although it is most common to find the cysts in the stool. *Giardia* inhabits the upper gastrointestinal tract and if stool microscopy is unhelpful it can be found in jejunal fluid or seen on jejunal biopsy. Damage to the mucosa is variable. The incubation period is about two weeks and symptoms may vary from lethargy, abdominal distension, anorexia and weight loss with offensive stools to frank diarrhoea and gross malabsorption. Treatment with Metronidazole is usually effective but stools should be checked 6–8 weeks after treatment to confirm satisfactory eradication.

# Question 1.4

This patient had severe discomfort from these ulcers but there were no systemic symptoms. Examination was normal but an iron deficiency anaemia was found.

1. Name four differential diagnoses.
2. Name three investigations which would most help to establish the diagnosis.

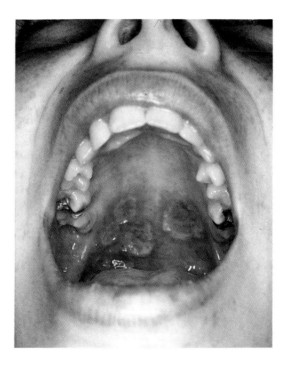

## Answer to question 1.4

1. Crohn's disease, ulcerative colitis, coeliac disease, Behçet's syndrome, pemphigus, pemphigoid, erythema multiforme and syphylis.
2. Small bowel enema, barium enema and small intestinal biopsy.

The presence of mouth ulcers with few systemic symptoms and an iron deficiency anaemia make a diagnosis of Crohn's disease or coeliac disease most likely. Mouth ulcers and iron deficiency are also found in ulcerative colitis but the patient would usually have had diarrhoea. The other conditions listed can be distinguished in most cases by the history, clinical examination and possibly biopsy of an ulcer.

If Crohn's disease is found in the gastrointestinal tract but is asymptomatic, oral iron plus local steroids to the mouth are the best initial treatment. Systemic steroids would be necessary if gastrointestinal disease became symptomatic. Mouth ulcers in coeliac disease usually heal when a gluten-free diet is adhered to.

# Question 1.5

This 70-year-old patient, who was otherwise well, developed poor vision.
**1.** What is the diagnosis?
**2.** What is the prognosis of the condition?

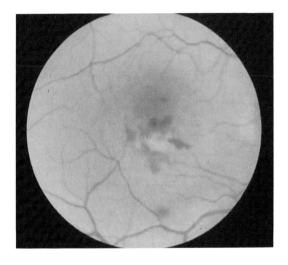

## Answer to question 1.5

1. Disciform degeneration of the macula.
2. Central vision becomes severely impaired.
   99% are registerable as partially sighted or blind within a year.


Senile macular degeneration is the most common cause of poor vision in the Western Hemisphere. It affects both sexes equally, usually occurring after the fifth decade. Two forms can be identified. The first is an atrophic form in which there is pigmentation in the macular area but no haemorrhage, exudate or scarring. The second, shown in this picture, is disciform macular degeneration in which there are degenerative changes at the level of Bruch's membrane which lead to thickening of that membrane and the formation of colloid bodies (drusen). In addition, new vessels arising from the choroid sheath invade through Bruch's membrane resulting in haemorrhage, retinal detachment and scarring.

85% of lesions are parafoveal if seen within two weeks of the initial symptom. Photocoagulation can be beneficial in these early stages where the lesion is adjacent to, rather than beneath the fovea centralis. Therefore, early recognition and referral to an ophthalmologist is essential.

# Question 1.6

What is the diagnosis?

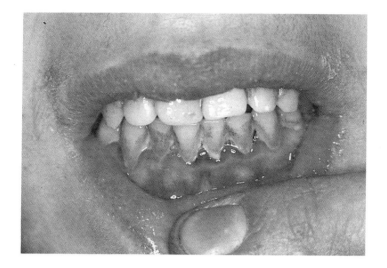

## Answer to question 1.6

Lead lines (plumbism).

Lead lines are deposits of lead acquired by either inhalation or ingestion. In children the lead may be ingested from toys painted with lead paint but in adults it is usually acquired from the burning of battery cases or drinking water from lead pipes. Patients may also complain of constipation, a metallic taste in the mouth or neuromuscular disorders such as foot drop. The diagnosis is confirmed by the finding of an increased serum lead and stippled red cells may be seen on the blood film. Bismuth ingestion may also give a similar line.

# Question 1.7

Why did this patient present with recurrent attacks of abdominal pain after meals?

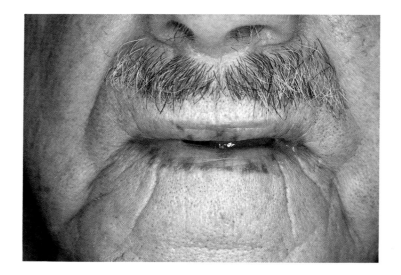

## Answer to question 1.7

Recurrent intussusception due to intestinal polyposis associated with the Peutz-Jeghers syndrome.

Mucocutaneous melanosis with gastrointestinal hamartomas (Peutz-Jeghers syndrome) is an autosomal dominant trait originally described by Peutz in 1921 and rediscovered by Jeghers et al in 1949. The oral pigmentation is due to increased melanin in the basal layer. The intestinal polyps may give rise to haematemesis, anaemia, intussusception, melaena or rectal bleeding depending on their location. Most commonly they are found in the jejunum and ileum and may rarely undergo malignant change.

# Question 1.8

What two conditions come to mind?
What other features would you look for?

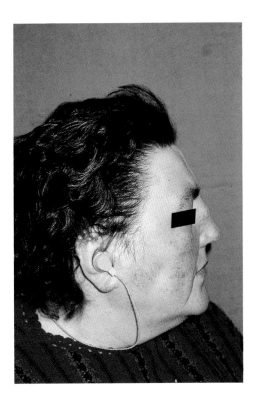

## Answer to question 1.8

Relapsing polychondritis or congenital syphilis.

This middle-aged woman shows a saddle-nose and has a hearing aid. She also has abnormal pinnae. Relapsing polychondritis is a rare condition which affects both sexes equally and may appear at any age. Its aetiology is unknown but it consists of recurrent attacks of tender inflammation of cartilage with its eventual destruction. It affects the nasal septum, pinnae, bridge of the nose and other cartilaginous structures. The patient may present to the rheumatologist with an asymmetrical sero-negative arthropathy. It may rarely also affect the aorta giving aortic dilatation and aortic valve regurgitation. A serious complication is involvement of the larynx and tracheal cartilaginous rings. Airways obstruction and stridor due to a floppy trachea are poor prognostic features. Deafness is due to collapse of the external auditory meatus. The diagnosis is often clinical although in an acute exacerbation one may see a raised ESR and a normochromic normocytic anaemia. Cartilage biopsy shows a vasculitis.

The differential diagnosis here is from congenital syphilis. The infection would be acquired in utero but late in pregnancy. The saddle-nose is only one of a large collection of other facial features including frontal bossing, poorly developed maxillae, corneal opacification and the rhagades which are scars at the corner of the mouth and nose due to early bacterial infection. Other confirmatory signs include the sabre tibia, optic atrophy and choroidoretinitis.

# Question 1.9

The patient presented with episodic attacks of wheezing; what is the diagnosis? What test would you do to confirm your suspicions?

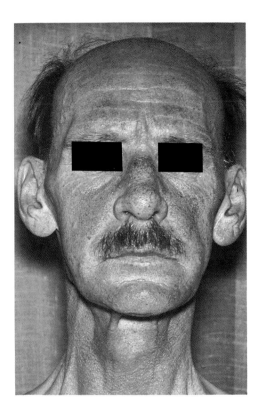

## Answer to question 1.9

Carcinoid syndrome. Urinary 5-hydroxy indole acetic acid (5HIAA) estimation.

The carcinoid syndrome may consist of flushing, telangiectasia, diarrhoea, valvular lesions and bronchoconstriction, although the presenting symptom may be very variable. The enterochromaffin tumour is derived from the embryonic foregut and may be present in the appendix, ileum, pancreas, stomach or bronchus and the intestinal varieties metastasise to the liver. Often the primary is small and undetectable. The tumour is slow-growing and life expectancy may be several years. Surgery to remove hepatic metastases may be helpful if these form the bulk of tumour and symptoms are severe despite medical therapy. Hepatic embolisation of tumour has been successful in experienced hands. Though the 5-HIAA may be elevated these tumours often secrete other vasoactive peptides and serotonin is not responsible for the majority of symptoms. Radiotherapy may be useful for bone pain but the tumour shows little response to it or chemotherapy.

# Question 1.10

1. What is the major clinical sign found in this condition?
2. What particular cellular analysis is a specific finding in this disease?

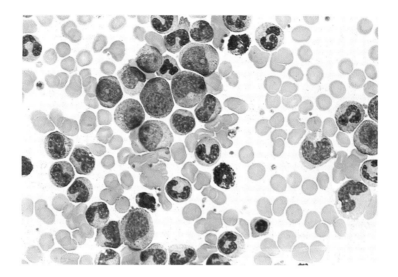

## Answer to question 1.10

**1.** Splenomegaly.
**2.** Chromosomal analysis for the Philadelphia Chromosome, a translocation of a part of chromosome 22 onto chromosome 9.

This is a blood film of a patient with chronic granulocytic leukaemia (CGL). Some patients with CGL present with acute symptoms such as abdominal pain from splenic infarction, evidence of haemorrhage or gout. Other patients present with chronic symptoms such as tiredness, malaise, weight loss or abdominal discomfort. The disease is discovered by chance in about 20% of patients. On examination, the spleen is usually found to be very large but may only just be palpable and the liver is also enlarged in most patients.

The diagnosis is established by finding splenomegaly, the characteristic blood film containing immature granulocytes, the cellular marrow with many immature cells, the Philadelphia chromosome and a low leucocyte alkaline phosphatase.

# Question 1.11

1. Name two abnormalities visible here.
2. Name three complications of this condition.

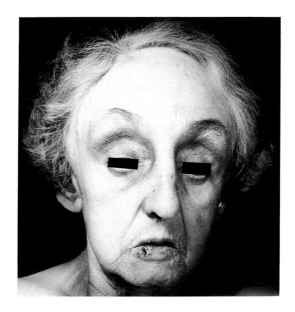

## Answer to question 1.11

1. Deafness, skull deformity.
2. Stress fractures.
   Nerve compression and platybasia.
   High output cardiac failure.
   Osteosarcoma.

Paget's disease is characterised by disorganised osteoclastic reabsorption and osteoblastic formation of bone. The matrix is laid down in a random fashion and mineralisation may also be defective. Pagetic bone is larger and more vascular than normal and is often deformed. Common sites of involvement are the axial skeleton (pelvis and spine). Complications include pain, deformity, fracture, high output cardiac failure, nerve deafness and cranial nerve compression. Paget's osteosarcoma is rare and occurs in less than 1% of patients. Serum biochemistry shows elevated alkaline phosphatase reflecting osteoblast activity. Calcium and phosphate are usually normal so an increase in plasma calcium suggests co-existent hyperparathyroidism but also may result from immobility. Therapy includes the use of calcitonin or diphosphanates if indicated.

## Question 1.12

This patient presented with dysphagia.
1. What is the cause of the dysphagia?
2. What is the mode of inheritance of the condition?

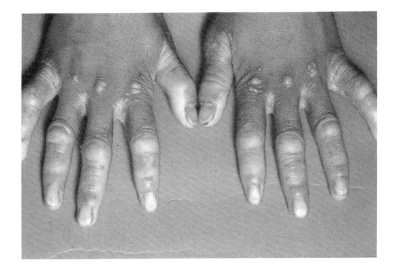

## Answer to question 1.12

**1.** Carcinoma of the oesophagus.
**2.** Autosomal dominant trait.


This is a rare skin disease known as tylosis. It is characterised by marked hyperkeratosis of the palms and soles; although changes may be seen on the dorsum of the hands as seen in this picture. It is inherited as an autosomal dominant character. In affected members of the family there can be up to a 45% chance of developing an oesophageal tumour. Members of the family without tylosis do not have an increased risk of developing this malignancy.

# Question 1.13

This patient who was generally well was found to have hypertension.
1. What is the abnormality in the picture shown here?
2. What is the prognosis with regard to visual acuity in this patient?

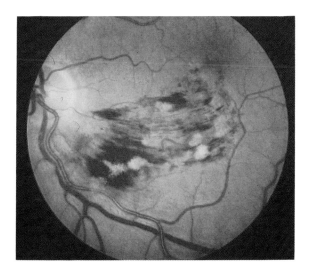

## Answer to question 1.13

**1.** Branch vein occlusion.
**2.** Visual loss is often severe in retinal vein thrombosis because of foveal capillary damage or macular oedema.

Diabetes mellitus and hypertension should be looked for in any patient found to have a retinal vein thrombosis. In addition, glaucoma and the hyperviscosity syndrome should be excluded. Visual loss is likely to remain in this patient because the macula is involved at the edge of the haemorrhage. Photocoagulation can help in such patients.

# Question 1.14

What abnormality is shown in this renal biopsy?

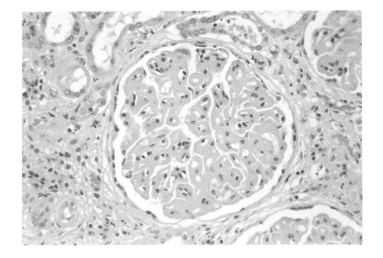

## Answer to question 1.14

Amyloid.

Recent studies have shown that this may be an immunocyte-related disease and biochemical analysis of the extracellular proteinaceous material has confirmed that the deposits are immunoglobulin fragments (usually portions of the light chain). It is suggested that in all types there is a monoclone producing either light chains or other forms of immunoglobulin and the stage or extent of the disease merely reflects the quantity of light chain present. Clinically the disease is still divided into primary or secondary either to chronic inflammation/infection (rheumatoid arthritis, osteomyelitis or bronchiectasis) or to a lymphoproliferative disorder (myeloma, Waldenström's macroglobulinaemia or non-Hodgkin's lymphoma).

There is often light chain excretion in the urine which may be obscured by the glomerular leak of protein with renal involvement. Nephrotic syndrome, renal vein thrombosis and progressive renal impairment may follow. Renal or cardiac involvement by amyloid is a poor prognostic sign.

# Question 1.15

1. What are the complications of this condition?
2. What is known about its mode of acquisition?

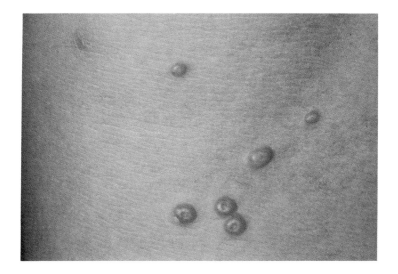

## Answer to question 1.15

1. Rarely conjunctivitis, keratitis and secondary infection.
2. Mode of infection from person to person is essentially unknown though it appears to be caught through contaminated water such as occurs in swimming pools.

*Molluscum contagiosum* is a benign DNA virus of the pox group. The incubation period is estimated to be between 2 and 7 weeks and most of the infections are probably acquired in swimming pools. It usually occurs in children and resolves within 2–4 months. However it may be seen in adults where sexually transmitted genital lesions can be found. The diagnosis can be confirmed by histology or stained smears of the central cores. Immunosuppressed individuals may get widespread lesions and if around the eye conjunctivitis and keratitis may occur or the lesion may become secondarily infected.

## Question 1.16

This patient complained of sudden onset of headache with vomiting.
1. What is the abnormality shown?
2. What sequence of investigations would you follow?
3. Where is the lesion?

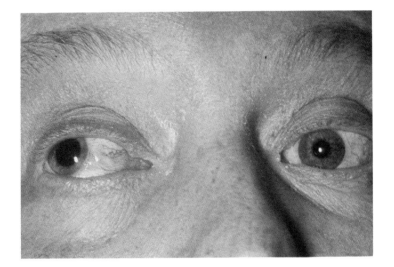

## Answer to question 1.16

**1.** Partial right third cranial nerve (oculomotor) palsy.
**2.** (a)  A computerised scan (CT).
     (b)  Lumbar puncture.
     (c)  Carotid angiography.
**3.** Posterior communicating artery.


The third cranial nerve supplies all the external ocular
muscles with the exception of the superior oblique and
lateral rectus. It also carries the parasympatheic
(constrictor) fibres of the iris. A partial third nerve palsy is
shown in this picture. A complete palsy produces a dilated
and unreactive pupil, complete ptosis and loss of upward,
downward and medial movement of the eye. This results in
the eye being deviated downwards and laterally. The history
given here suggests a subarachnoid haemorrhage which in
combination with a third nerve palsy should always indicate
a posterior communicating artery aneurysm. When a
subarachnoid haemorrhage is suspected with focal
neurological signs as in this patient, it is preferable to carry
out a computerised tomographic scan in the first instance. If
CT scanning is not available lumbar puncture would confirm
the presence of blood in the CSF. Carotid angiography
confirms the presence of an aneurysm in 80% of patients,
but early diagnosis and surgical intervention may be
inadvisable in patients with focal neurological defects.

# Question 1.17

1. What is this preparation?
2. What abnormal cells are present?
3. List three causes of this condition.

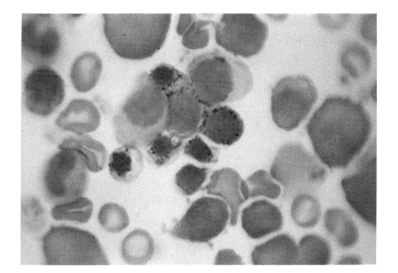

# Answer to question 1.17

1. Bone marrow preparation stained for iron.
2. Normoblasts are present with increased iron around the nucleus. These are ring sideroblasts and are diagnostic of sideroblastic anaemia.
3. The sideroblastic anaemias may be congenital (X-linked) or acquired. The acquired form may be primary (idiopathic) or secondary to drugs (e.g. isoniazid and chloramphenicol), alcohol, lead, malabsorption, myeloproliferative disorders, leukaemias, or secondary carcinoma.

The sideroblastic anaemias are characterised by severe dyserythropoiesis with marked iron loading of red cell precursors and in some cases widespread haemosiderosis. Excess iron is situated in the mitochondria lying in a circle around the nucleus of the red cell precursors giving the name ring sideroblasts to these cells. The aetiology of the condition is unknown, but is probably an underlying abnormality of haemoglobin synthesis. In some of the acquired forms, specific mitochondrial toxins can be implicated.

Clinical and haematological features of the sideroblastic anaemias depend upon the aetiology. In the congenital form mainly males are affected and there is a dimorphic blood picture with extreme hypochromia, reduced MCH and MCV. The platelets and white cells are normal and there is frequently mild splenomegaly with marrow hyperplasia showing a large percentage of ring sideroblasts. The acquired forms tend to affect both sexes, splenomegaly is unusual, and although a dimorphic blood picture may be present the MCV is often normal or increased. Platelets may be reduced.

Diagnosis is made on the basis of a dimorphic blood picture with normochromic and hypochromic cells, followed by bone marrow examination looking for ring sideroblasts. A careful search for an underlying cause should be carried out. Pyridoxine treatment may be successful but therapy is otherwise supportive.

# Question 1.18

Why might this patient present (a) to an ophthalmologist? (b) to a cardiologist?

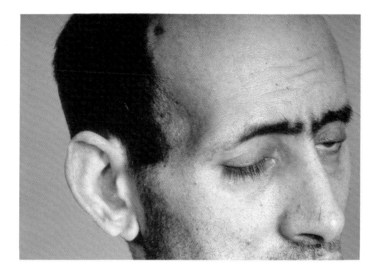

## Answer to question 1.18

(a) Progressive deterioration in vision due to sub-capsular or senile cataracts.
(b) Atrial arrhythmias associated with dystrophic heart disease.


Dystrophia myotonica is inherited as a mendelian dominant trait and the features are muscle myotonia, cataracts, mental retardation, testicular atrophy and frontal alopecia. The myotonia is often best demonstrated after periods of inactivity or on percussion (percussion myotonia) followed by slow relaxation which may be the first physical sign. The dull expressionless face with a furrowed forehead is an attempt to compensate for the ptosis. Frontal baldness is seen both in men and women. The testicular atrophy results in sterility in men but infertility is rare in women. The heart may be affected giving rise to atrial arrhythmias and the oesophagus may be dilated. The brain is often small. The diagnosis may be made by the EMG finding of after potentials.

# Question 1.19

1. What is the diagnosis?
2. Give three pieces of information that would help to confirm the diagnosis.

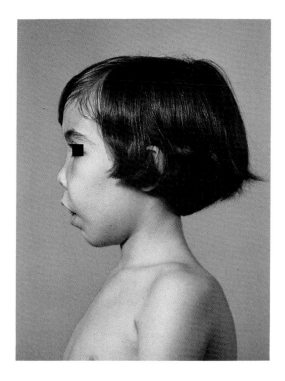

## Answer to question 1.19

**1.** β-Thalassaemia major.
**2.** (a) Racial background.
   (b) Blood count and film.
   (c) Haemoglobin electrophoresis.

β-Thalassaemia major (Cooley's anaemia) is inherited as an autosomal dominant trait. The disorder is found in countries bordering the Mediterranean and in a broad band extending east through the Middle East and Indian subcontinent to South East Asia. It is also found in parts of West Africa. Symptoms of severe anaemia occur together with jaundice, leg ulcers and cholelithiasis. Massive splenomegaly is common. Hyperactivity of the bone marrow causes thickening of the cranial bones and malar eminences. Pathological fractures are common.

   The anaemia is severe with microcytosis and hypochromia and there is a high reticulocyte count. The film is characteristic showing large numbers of nucleated erythroblasts, target cells, microcytic hypochromic red cells and punctate basophilia. Haemoglobin electrophoresis reveals high levels of haemoglobin F ranging from 30–90% of the total. There is no haemoglobin A and the remainder of the haemoglobin consists of $A_2$.

# Question 1.20

1. What is the diagnosis?
2. What is the most common cause?

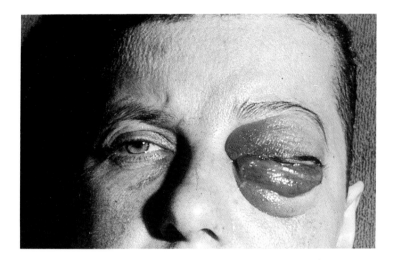

## Answer to question 1.20

**1.** Cavernous sinus thrombophlebitis.
**2.** Occulonasal infection.


The most common infecting agent is a coagulase-negative staphylococcus which has infected either the eye, the nose or the face. The clinical syndrome consists of orbital oedema, chemosis, venous congestion and an ophthalmoplegia. The thrombophelbitis may spread to the opposite side as well via the circular sinus. The treatment is with suitable antibiotics and the use of anticoagulants is disputed.

# Paper 2

Paper 2

# Question 2.1

How would you confirm the diagnosis?

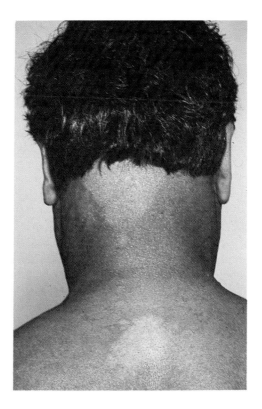

## Answer to question 2.1

Slit-smear examination of the skin lesion or skin biopsy.

The response to *Mycobacterium leprae* infection may vary from mild (tuberculoid) to a severe anergic response (lepromatous) with a negative lepromin test dependent on the hosts ability to generate specific cell mediated immunity. Often the mycobacteria can be demonstrated in a slit-smear preparation and skin biopsy shows the granulomata concentrated around the schwann cells. Often the patients present with sensory disturbance before the skin lesions. These may vary from a few millimeters to large areas of hypopigmented or depigmented skin. In the anergic lepromatous type damage and infiltration of the nerves is a late feature.

The Lepromin test is performed by injecting intradermal autoclaved suspension of *M. leprae*. It is read at 48 h (Fernandez reaction) and 3–5 weeks (Mitsuda reaction). The latter gives an accurate assessment of specific cell mediated immunity. The test is positive in tuberculoid and negative in lepromatous disease but is not diagnostic as false positives occur.

# Question 2.2

1. What abnormalities are present in this bone-marrow preparation and what is the most likely diagnosis?
2. Name three adverse prognostic features of this condition.

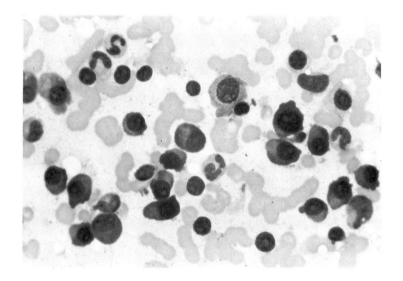

# Answer to question 2.2

1. Atypical plasma cells are the predominant cell type shown. They have an eccentric nucleus, prominent Golgi zone and deep blue cytoplasm. This is consistent with a diagnosis of multiple myeloma. Bi- or multi-nucleated plasma cells (not present here) may also be seen.

   The diagnostic triad necessary to confirm this condition is:
   (a) osteolytic bone lesions
   (b) atypical plasma cells in the marrow
   (c) homogeneous band of abnormal globulin migrating in the gamma or beta zones.
   Often light chains are present in the urine.

2. The MRC criteria defining poor prognosis at diagnosis includes a haemoglobin of less than 7.5 g/dl, a blood urea above 10 mmol/l, and physical activity restricted through symptoms.

## Question 2.3

This patient consulted her GP regarding a sore throat.
1. What is this lesion?
2. What sites may be affected?

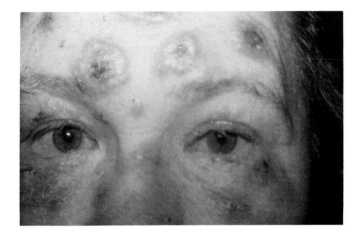

## Answer to question 2.3

1. Erythema multiforme.
2. Face, hands, flexor aspects of the forearms and knees, mucous membranes and conjunctivae.


Erythema multiforme is a polymorphic skin reaction to a variety of stimuli showing annular red lesions with a purple centre which in time show colour changes similar to a bruise (so called 'iris' lesions). When severe these lesions show vesicle or even bullous formation. Mucous membranes may be involved and may be shed leaving a raw red surface to which shreds of mucosa still adhere. These signs may be accompanied by a severe constitutional disturbance with pyrexia – the so-called Stevens-Johnson syndrome.

Causes of this condition include:

(a) Viral infections, particularly herpes simplex
(b) *Strep. haemolyticus, Mycoplasma pneumoniae*
(c) Drugs, particularly sulphonamides and barbituates
(d) Leukaemia
(e) SLE.

Treatment tends to be symptomatic, involving anti-pruritic agents (both topical and systemic) and anti-viral agents if the syndrome was precipitated by herpes. Although systemic steroid therapy has been advocated in this condition it has not been shown to shorten the course but may be of value in individuals with severe constitutional disturbance.

# Question 2.4

What does this heart show?

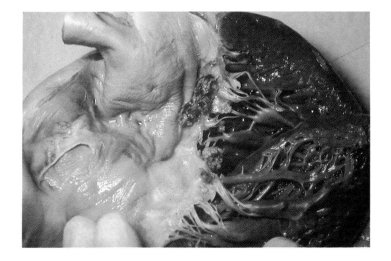

## Answer to question 2.4

Vegetations on the mitral valve of bacterial endocarditis.

Bacteria will colonise an already compromised valve and previously this was mostly due to rheumatic valvular disease and congenital heart disease. The pattern is however changing in that infection is occurring with more diverse organisms on prosthetic valves. In the past up to 90% of SBE organisms were of the *Streptococcus viridans* type but now this figure has fallen to less than 50%. The incidence of micro-aerophilic and Lancefield group D streptococci (*Strep. bovis, Strep. faecalis*) has increased. Once established the patient may present with pyrexia, increasing heart failure or embolisation. Clinically one would search for splinter haemorrhages, Oslers nodes, Janeway lesions, Roth spots, microscopic haematuria and slight splenomegaly. Cardiac ultrasound is a useful diagnostic tool but blood cultures remain essential for the culture of the organism.

In acute bacterial endocarditis the organism is usually *Staphylococcus aureus, Strep. pneumoniae* or gram negative bacteria. Infection occurs in up to 50% of patients on previously normal valves. Abscess formation and rapidly deteriorating heart failure result in a poor prognosis.

# Question 2.5

This young patient presented with poor vision, general malaise and a sore throat.

1. What single investigation would you do to confirm your diagnosis?
2. Name two ways in which this condition may be acquired.

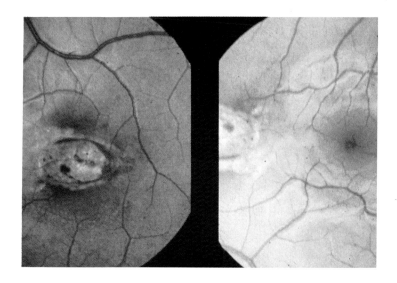

## Answer to question 2.5

**1.** A serological test for toxoplasmosis.
**2.** Congenital infection, from eating uncooked meat and from close contact with cats.

Toxoplasmosis is caused by a protozoan, *Toxoplasma gondii*. It is a common cause of chorioretinitis. The incidence varies from country to country but about 50% of 70-year-olds have serological evidence of previous infection in the UK. The acquired infection usually resembles glandular fever and in the great majority of cases complete recovery occurs in weeks or months. A few patients develop myocarditis or rarely encephalitis. These complications are more common in immunocompromised patients. Congenital infection may occur being particularly serious during the first trimester when serious congenital abnormalities may develop.

Ocular toxoplasmosis is nearly always present after a congenital infection and is a common cause of chorioretinitis in patients with the acquired disease. It affects mostly the posterior pole and the fovea centralis may be destroyed. Initially there is acute chorioretinitis followed by resolution to pigmented scars as seen in this picture. The organism may remain as a dormant cyst.

# Question 2.6

Name two drugs that may cause this condition.

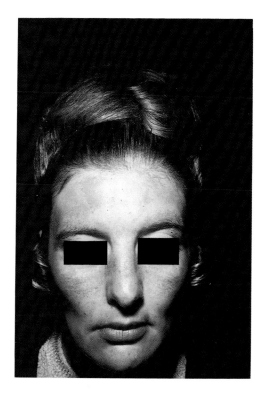

## Answer to question 2.6

Oral contraceptives, sodium phenytoin.

Hypermelanosis (chloasma) is seen most commonly in pregnancy and in those on oral contraceptives. It is also seen rarely in patients taking phenytoin and others with ovarian tumours. The macules appear most commonly on the face and in exposed areas but their aetiology is unknown. The serum MSH level is normal and it has been suggested that it may be due to an alteration in the balance between oestrogen and progesterone.

# Question 2.7

This patient presented to a hospital while on a camping holiday, the lesions rapidly resolved on returning home.

1. Why are these lesions found on the legs?
2. What two complications can be life-threatening in this group of disorders?
3. What single investigation would you do to confirm the diagnosis in the familial form of this condition?

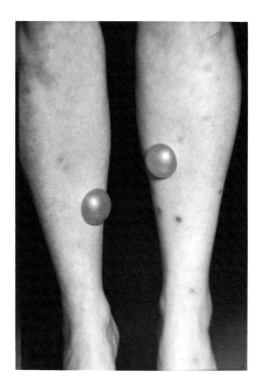

## Answer to question 2.7

1. These lesions are caused by insect bites most commonly found on the lower legs.
2. (i) Anaphylactic shock.
   (ii) Angio-oedema of the upper respiratory tract.
   (iii) Disseminated intravascular coagulation.
3. $C_1$ esterase inhibitor level in serum.


This patient is suffering from papular urticaria. The life threatening conditions are not common with papular urticaria but are found more frequently with other causes of urticaria such as bee stings and various drugs. Familial angio-oedema, inherited as an autosomal dominant trait, should be suspected if there is a family history. This is frequently complicated by recurrent abdominal pain. A low level of $C_1$ esterase inhibitor is found in the serum of these patients.

## Question 2.8

This patient has complained of arthritis, conjunctivitis and one other symptom.
1. What was that other symptom?
2. With what condition are these symptoms associated?
3. It may follow some other conditions: name one.

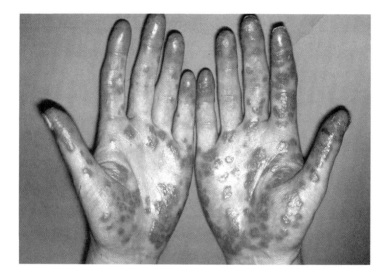

## Answer to question 2.8

1. Urethritis – either gonococcal or non-gonococcal.
2. Reiter's syndrome.
3. Enteric infections, such as bacillary dysentry, salmonellosis and yersiniosis.

Keratoderma blenorrhagica is the characteristic skin lesion of Reiter's syndrome. It usually affects the soles of the feet but may also occur on the dorsum of the feet, the penis, palms, scalp and trunk. The lesions usually but not always resolve in about a month. Reiter's syndrome is a condition of uncertain aetiology characterised by seronegative polyarthropathy, conjunctivitis and non-specific urethritis. The condition was originally described after attacks of dysentery and only later associated with sexually transmitted urethritis. With both these aetiologies of Reiter's syndrome there is a close association with the presence of HLA-B27.

## Question 2.9

This patient presented in adolescence with difficulty in walking.

1. What deformity is commonly associated with this disorder?
2. What abnormality may be found in the upper limbs?
3. What is the pathological lesion found in these patients?

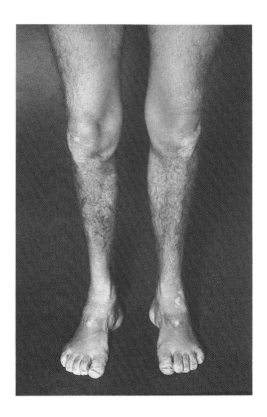

## Answer to question 2.9

1. Pes cavus.
2. Peripheral motor and sensory neuropathy may be found in the hands.
3. Segmental demyelination of peripheral nerves.

Hereditary motor and sensory polyneuropathy (Charcot-Marie-Tooth disease, Peroneal muscular atrophy) is usually transmitted by dominant inheritance. It is a relatively common disorder characterised by weakness and atrophy of the muscles in the lower legs, particularly the peroneal muscles. The small muscles of the hands may also be involved. A peripheral sensory neuropathy in both the lower and upper limbs is common. Two types of the disease are now described. In type I, usually beginning in the first ten years of life, pes cavus and scoliosis are common and nerve conduction is severely affected. The type II form usually begins in adolescence but may not begin until late adult life. Pes cavus is less common and nerve conduction less severely reduced. Diagnosis is established by the clinical findings, including the family history aided if necessary by nerve conduction studies. Histologically there is demyelination and/or axonal degeneration of the peripheral nerves. The patients usually remain active for many years and have a normal life span.

## Question 2.11

This patient is attempting to oppose the palms of his hands.
1. What drug might he be taking?
2. What is the explanation for this appearance?

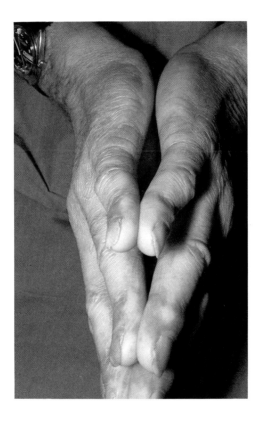

## Answer to question 2.11

1. Insulin.
2. Limited joint mobility or tendon contractures seen in diabetes mellitus.

Only recently has this feature been recognised in diabetes. They appear to develop abnormal collagen around joints and in tendons which may produce joint contracture and tight waxy skin over the dorsum of the hands. This results in a failure to be able to completely extend the fingers. The patients are usually insulin dependent and it has been suggested that this is more common in those with proliferative retinopathy and nephropathy.

Dupuytren's contractures associated with alcohol and phenytoin characteristically tend to affect the ring and/or the little finger.

# Question 2.12

This patient had tremor and dysarthria. His right eye had been injured during childhood.
1. What is the diagnosis?
2. Excluding the abnormal right eye name three other abnormal physical signs present in this picture.
3. The patient was diagnosed when he was 62 years old: please comment.

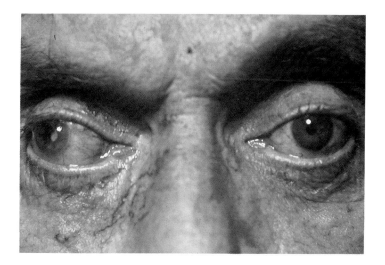

## Answer to question 2.12

**1.** Wilson's disease.
**2.** Jaundice, spider naevi, unilateral Kayser-Fleischer ring.
**3.** This is an exceptionally old age for a patient to be diagnosed as having Wilson's disease.

Wilson's disease should be suspected in all patients with unexplained neurological, liver or psychiatric disease particularly if the patient is under 40 years old. This is a very rare case with the diagnosis not being made until the age of 62. It is very important that the disease is recognised early as treatment with chelating agents usually results in clinical improvement. The diagnosis is established by finding a low serum copper, low caeruloplasmin, high urinary copper, high liver copper and Kayser-Fleisher rings on slit lamp examination. All of these tests may be normal in exceptional circumstances but a combination of the clinical features and investigation results will establish the diagnosis.

This patient is unique in being found to have a striking left sided Kayser-Fleischer ring with no ring in the right eye. It is thought that this may be due to the abnormal flow of aqueous humor in the damaged eye preventing the deposition of copper in the cornea.

# Question 2.13

1. What is this lesion?
2. Name three other genital lesions from which it must be differentiated.

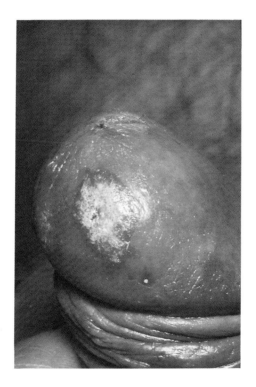

## Answer to question 2.13

**1.** Chancre of primary syphilis.
**2.** Genital herpes.
Drug eruption (Stevens-Johnson syndrome).
Chancroid.
(Also consider infected traumatic sores, scabies, Behcet's syndrome, granuloma inguinale and lymphogranuloma venereum.)

The chancre of primary syphilis usually appears 2–6 weeks (range of 9–90 days) after the initial infection and heals within 2–6 weeks. It starts as a small painless papule which rapidly ulcerates. The lesion is solitary, and indurated and in heterosexual men is found most commonly on the coronal sulcus, glans, inner surface of the prepuce, mouth, lips or fingers. In homosexual men it may also be found in the anal canal. In heterosexual women the vulva, labia and cervix are common sites. Regional lymphadenopathy is usual several days after the appearance of the lesion. *Treponema pallidum* can often be demonstrated on dark field illumination of serum taken from the chancre or associated lymph nodes.

The differential diagnoses are genital herpes, drug eruptions and chancroid. Herpetic lesions tend to be intensely irritative whilst drug eruptions are usually multifocal often involving the mouth and face. Chancroid occurs mainly in the tropics and is a painful superfical soft lesion associated with supurative adenitis.

# Question 2.14

1. What is the inheritance of this condition?
2. What is the proposed biochemical abnormality?

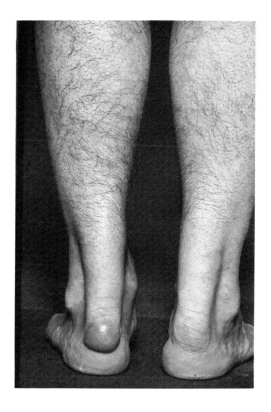

# Answer to question 2.14

**1.** Autosomal dominant trait.
**2.** Deficiency of cell receptors for low density lipoprotein.


Tendon xanthomata are associated with familial hypercholesterolaemia, an autosomal dominant trait with an excess of low density lipoprotein or beta lipoprotein in blood. Familial hypercholesterolaemia occurs in 1 in 200 to 500 of the population. Goldstein & Brown in 1975 showed that this condition was associated with a defect or deficiency of cell receptors for low density lipoprotein. Homozygotes usually appear with xanthomata as children or even at birth. They have a predisposition to ischaemic heart disease which usually results in death before the age of 30. 50% of heterozygotes present with xanthomata by the same age.

# Question 2.15

This patient complained of recurrent headaches.
1. What is the diagnosis?
2. What would you expect to find when examining the visual fields of this patient?

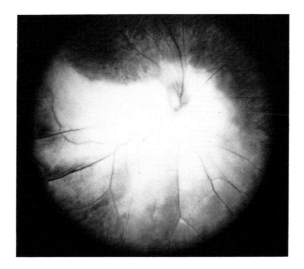

## Answer to question 2.15

**1.** Myelinated nerve fibres which is a normal variant.
**2.** Normal visual fields.

The optic nerve fibres are normally myelinated to the lamina cribrosa as the nerve passes through the sclera at the back of the eye. Occasionally the myelination extends into the eye giving the appearances seen in this picture. The visual fields are normal and there are no long-term consequences. The headache was unrelated to this finding.

# Question 2.16

1. What physical signs does this patient show?
2. What is the diagnosis?
3. What two tests might you perform?

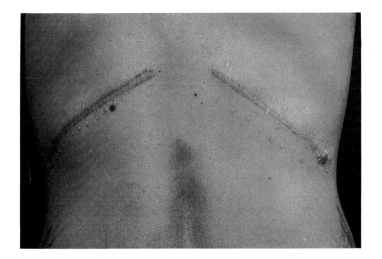

## Answer to question 2.16

1. Bilateral adrenalectomy scars for Cushing's syndrome.
   Increased skin pigmentation.
2. Nelson's syndrome
3. Serum ACTH.
   Computerised tomography (CT) scan of the pituitary
   fossa.

Treatment of Cushing's syndrome by sub-total
adrenalectomy was unsatisfactory and subsequently total
bilateral adrenalectomy was performed. However, 20–30%
develop Nelson's syndrome following this procedure due to
very high ACTH levels which stimulate melanin production
by melanocytes leading to the skin pigmentation.

The excessive production of ACTH is often as a result of
the release of a pituitary adenoma from the negative
feedback by high levels of circulating cortisol. A CT scan
may reveal the adenoma and, if suitable, a transphenoidal
hypophysectomy would be the treatment of choice.

## Question 2.17

This patient recently returned from a holiday in Spain.
1. What is the diagnosis?
2. How may it be confirmed?
3. Name three drugs associated with this disorder.

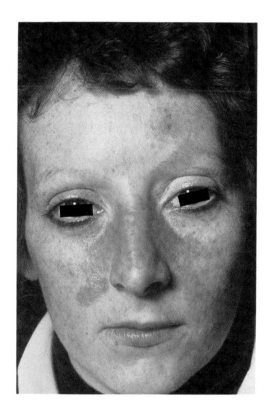

## Answer to question 2.17

1. Systemic lupus erythematosis (SLE).
2. Detection of anti-DNA antibody.
3. Drugs that induce SLE – hydrallazine, isoniazid, anti-convulsants and procainamide.

Systemic lupus erythematosis (SLE) is a multi-system connective tissue disorder. Humoral antibodies against double stranded DNA, nucleic and cytoplasmic cellular components are seen. These together with the presence of a wide range of organ specific and viral antibodies has led to the suggestion that there may be a defect in T-cell suppressor function in this condition. Such a defect would result in failure to eliminate antigens (e.g. viruses) and failure to suppress B-cell activity with excessive humoral antibody production. Major clinical manifestations of SLE include: musculo-skeletal problems (95%), cutaneous manifestations (81%), fever (77%), neuropsychiatric disorders (59%), renal (53%), pulmonary (48%) or cardiac involvement (38%).

Drug-induced lupus is very much less common than SLE. The incidence of a positive ANF is much higher than in frank clinical lupus. The clinical features when they do emerge resemble those of SLE but pulmonary involvement is common. DNA antibodies are usually absent or low in drug induced LE. In patients with known SLE some drugs such as penicillamine and the oral contraceptive may produce an exacerbation.

# Question 2.18

1. What is the diagnosis in this patient?
2. What feature seen in this picture helps to define the diagnosis more precisely?

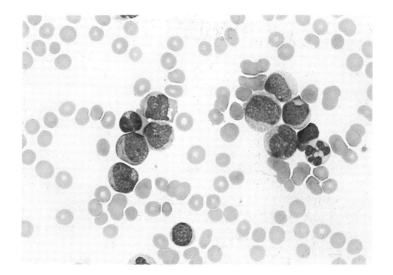

## Answer to question 2.18

**1.** Acute myeloblastic leukaemia.
**2.** The presence of Auer rods indicate a myeloid or myelomonocytic leukaemia.

The clinical features and examination of a blood film for blast cells usually establishes the diagnosis of acute leukaemia. However, microscopic examination of the bone marrow is essential to confirm the diagnosis. Chromosome and immunological studies of the bone marrow may also be helpful. Acute myeloid or myelomonoblastic leukaemias are characterised by specific morphological characteristics and in particular Auer rods in the cytoplasm of the myeloblasts when one of the Romanowsky stains is used. The Auer rods are probably composed of several of the specific granules fused together. Further more detailed subclassification, known as the FAB classification is now used, which identifies six groups of acute non-lymphoblastic and three groups of lymphoblastic leukaemias.

# Question 2.19

What are these lesions?

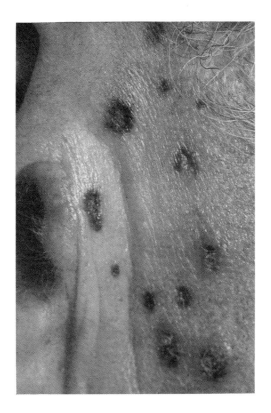

## Answer to question 2.19

Malignant melanoma with satellite lesions.

Malignant melanoma can be of various descriptive types –
nodular, superficial spreading or lentiga maligna. It may
vary in colour from black to having no pigment (amelanotic
melanoma). Lentiga melanoma occurs mainly on the face of
elderly persons and begins as a tan-coloured macule which
grows and darkens to form a black nodule.

Most melanomas arise from naevi. In a few patients with
metastatic melanoma large amounts of tyrosine oxidation
products made in the tumour reach the skin and are
converted to melanin. The patient first acquires the slate
grey colour similar to that seen in argyria and later becomes
intensely brown or black. Melanuria in which tyrosine
oxidation products are excreted in the urine become
oxidised to melanin giving the urine a dark colour.

Common sites of metastases include the liver, retina and
bones. Treatment is unsatisfactory but at the present
consists of wide excision of the primary lesion, with
chemotherapy and radiotherapy for symptomatic relief of
bone pain.

# Question 2.20

1. What abnormalities can be seen?
2. What is the underlying lesion?

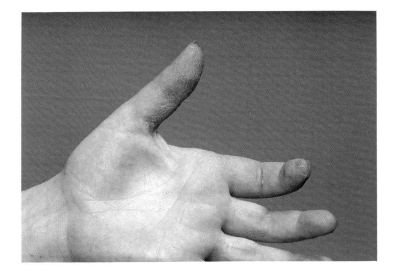

## Answer to question 2.20

1. Trophic skin changes over the dermatome of $C_6$ and some wasting of the thenar emminence.
2. There are three possible diagnoses for the abnormalities shown in this picture:
   (a) Partial median nerve lesion.
   (b) $C_6$ sensory root and $T_1$ motor root lesion.
   (c) $C_6$ sensory root lesion with wasting of the thenar eminence due to disuse.


The trophic skin changes seen in this picture are confined to the distribution of $C_6$. The skin changes would also involve the middle finger and lateral side of the ring finger if a complete median nerve palsy was present. All three of the above diagnoses were considered in this patient but no evidence of median nerve or $T_1$ root damage was found and the skin over the thumb and index finger was very tender. Therefore, a diagnosis of an isolated $C_6$ lesion was made with thenar wasting resulting from disuse.

# Paper 3

# Question 3.1

1. What is the most common initial sign in this disorder?
2. What is this condition?
3. What is the single most important part of the management of this condition?

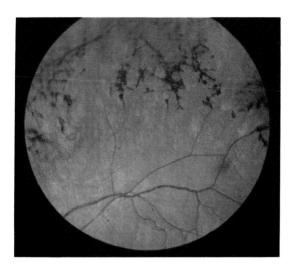

# Answer to question 3.1

1. Night blindness.
2. Retinitis pigmentosa.
3. A family study of the inheritance with appropriate genetic advice being given to the family.

Retinitis pigmentosa is a disorder in which the photoreceptors, primarily the rods, atrophy. It is a hereditary disorder which may be transmitted by autosomal dominant, autosomal recessive or sex-linked inheritance. Night blindness is usually the first sign due to the initial damage to the rods. There is classically a ring scotoma to begin with but this progresses, with the cones becoming involved, until vision is lost completely. The earliest ophthalmoscopic signs are the black pigment dots looking like 'bone spicules'. As the disease progresses the disc looks waxy and the retinal vessels become attenuated. It is thought that bright light may accelerate the process so this is avoided when possible. A study of the pattern of inheritance in each family affected should be done and appropriate genetic counselling should be undertaken.

# Question 3.2

1. What is this lesion?
2. Why is it important to diagnose?
3. Name another place where this lesion may be found.

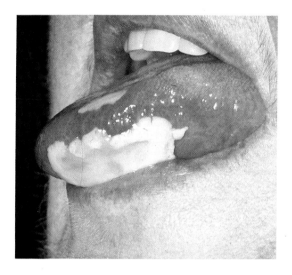

# Answer to question 3.2

**1.** Leukoplakia.
**2.** It can be premalignant.
**3.** In the anal region, lower rectum or vulva.

Leukoplakia is found in the mouth as shown in this picture and in the vulva. Rarely it may be in the perianal region and lower rectum. It is characterised by white plaques which consist of hyperkeratinised layers of squamous epithelium. Many factors have been implicated in the aetiology of oral leukoplakia including smoking, alcohol, poor teeth or poorly fitting dentures, spicy foods, syphilitic glossitis and *Candida albicans*.

Oral leukoplakia can usually be recognised on clinical examination but may appear in small patches on inflamed mucosa or may be brown in patients who smoke. It should be biopsied and if possible removed as it can become malignant. Causative irritants such as those mentioned above should cease to be used and poor teeth or dentures should be corrected. Careful follow-up of these patients is essential.

## Question 3.3

This patient with diabetes mellitus presented to the clinic complaining of palpitations.
1. What is the diagnosis?
2. To what are his symptoms attributable?

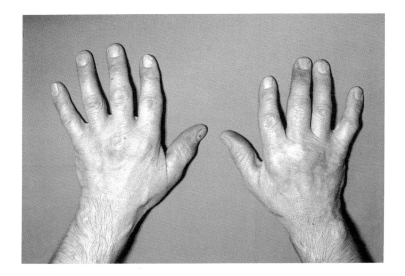

## Answer to question 3.3

1. Haemochromatosis.
2. Cardiac and pancreatic involvement leading to atrial fibrillation and diabetes.

Primary haemochromatosis is a genetically transmitted inborn error of iron absorption leading to severe iron overload. Heterozygotes may show only mild degrees and only become symptomatic if other factors – such as excessive alcohol intake and iron therapy – are superimposed. Clinical features include:
(a) Diabetes mellitus (80% of patients)
(b) Cardiac arrhythmias and heart failure (15%)
(c) Cirrhosis and occasionally hepatoma
(d) Skin pigmentation ('bronze diabetes')
(e) Arthropathy (50%) which usually involves the second and third metacarpo-phalangeal joints. Any of the small joints may be involved with swelling and deformity. Ulnar deviation does not occur.

# Question 3.4

1. What is this preparation?
2. What abnormalities are present?
3. Which type of disease is seen here?

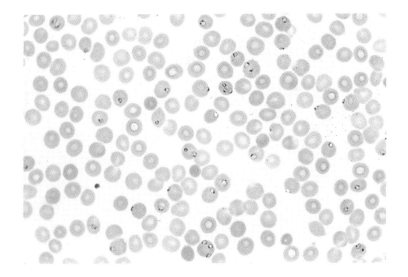

## Answer to question 3.4

**1.** Peripheral blood film.
**2.** Red cell inclusions are present – malarial parasites.
**3.** Falciparum malaria.

The presence of multiply infected erythrocytes with accole (peripheral) forms are indicative of falciparum malaria. Other criteria suggestive of this diagnosis include a predominance of small ring forms, double nuclei and the diagnostic crescent-shaped gametocytes. In addition, if more than 5% of red blood cells are infected falciparum should be suspected.

Once malarial parasites are identified on a blood film, the most important distinction to be made is between falciparum malaria and the other types, as all other forms may initially be treated with chloroquine. Chloroquine resistance to falciparum malaria has now emerged in several areas of the world including East Africa, Asia-east of Pakistan, South America and Panama. Alternative treatments to chloroquine or amodiaquine include pyrimethamine combined with quinine sulphate and a sulphonamide. The parasitaemia should be followed with twice daily blood films for 48 hours. No asexual parasites should be detected in smears 4–5 days after starting treatment. The gametocytes persist for weeks and do not indicate failed treatment.

# Question 3.5

This patient remained in this position and was unresponsive to painful stimuli.
1. What is the diagnosis?
2. What is the main differential diagnosis?

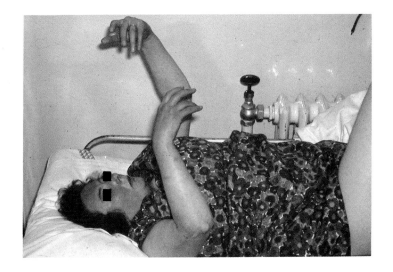

## Answer to question 3.5

**1.** Catatonic schizophrenia.
**2.** Hysteria.

Catatonic schizophrenia appears in two forms, stupor (as seen here) and excitement. There is usually a prodromal period when the patient gradually loses contact with the environment. Hallucinations, pursing or protrusion of the lips (schnauzkrampf), negativism or automatic obedience may all occur. In severe cases stupor may supervene when the patient may remain for hours in an unusual posture. Despite being in this state the patient may later recall all that happened. Excitement may precede or follow the stupor and can be difficult to distinguish from acute mania. However, in catatonic excitement, behaviour is purposeless, speech is incoherent, behaviour is often negativistic, hallucinations are almost invariable and it is difficult to establish rapport with the patient. Phenothiazines or butyrophenones are the mainstay of treatment. However, electroconvulsive therapy (ECT) may be useful in the stuporous or excitable state.

# Question 3.6

What does this pathology specimen show?

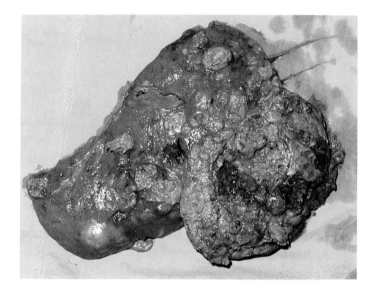

## Answer to question 3.6

Cirrhosis of the liver and a primary liver cell carcinoma (hepatoma).

Cirrhosis has many causes but the end result is the consequence of liver cell necrosis, fibrosis and regenerative nodule formation with eventual hepatic decompensation and portal hypertension. The development of a hepatoma should be suspected if weight loss, pain or a rapid deterioration in liver function occurs in a patient with cirrhosis as 80% of patients with this tumour have a pre-existing cirrhotic liver. High levels of alpha-fetoprotein of more than 1000 ng/ml are highly suggestive of this complication. Lower levels above the normal range may be found in active cirrhosis. The diagnosis, once suspected, may be substantiated by ultrasound, CT scan, radioisotope scan or arteriography and percutaneous liver biopsy is often performed for histological confirmation. Resection of the tumour is rarely feasible because of the cirrhosis and treatment has been either by chemotherapy or by tumour embolisation through a hepatic artery catheter. The prognosis is poor.

# Question 3.7

Name three physical signs.
    What is the diagnosis and give one other cause of the nail changes?

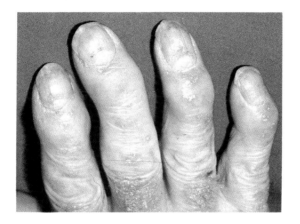

## Answer to question 3.7

Psoriasis with arthropathy and nail changes. Chronic eczema or patients with extensive alopecia areata may also show pitted nails.

Nail changes occur in up to 50% of psoriatic patients and the changes are rarely absent in patients with psoriatic arthropathy. The characteristic nail pits are also found in chronic eczema and patients with extensive alopecia arreata and therefore are not specific for psoriasis. Onycholysis and subungual hyperkeratosis with lifting the nail bed are also frequently seen. The arthropathy of psoriasis is usually limited to single joints of the hands or feet (70%) but 15% get a sero-negative rheumatoid-like pattern and the sacro-iliac joints may also be involved. The X-ray appearances of the joints show erosion but unlike rheumatoid the joint space is preserved. Cysts are present near the joint surface eventually giving the 'pencil in cup' appearance.

## Question 3.8

The patient presented with a progressive skin lesion which he had had for 4 weeks. Apart from a skin biopsy which showed non-specific changes what would be your next two investigations?

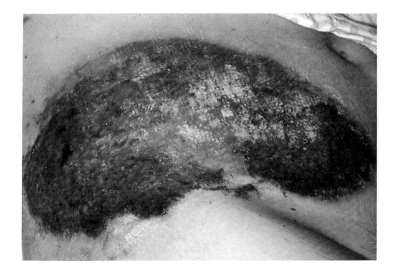

## Answer to question 3.8

Sigmoidoscopy and rectal biopsy, barium enema.

Pyoderma gangrenosa begins as a lesion with a central necrotic portion surrounded by a violaceous hue. It is most commonly associated with ulcerative colitis and Crohn's disease but also occurs in rheumatoid arthritis and various dysproteinaemias. Trauma may precipitate a new lesion and only rarely do the skin lesions precede the bowel symptoms. Its histological appearance is non-specific and it has been suggested that it may be an auto-sensitisation phenomenon similar to a Schwartzmann reaction as patients with pyoderma gangrenosa will also reject autologous skin grafts.

# Question 3.9

1. What is this condition?
2. What is it caused by?
3. What is the best treatment?

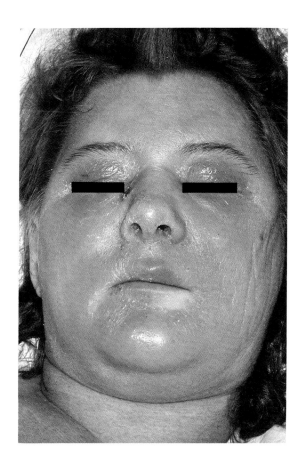

## Answer to question 3.9

**1.** Erysipelas.
**2.** Group A streptococci.
**3.** Benzyl penicillin.

The appearance of erysipelas is usually characteristic. It tends to occur later in life than the other group A streptococcal diseases which are found mainly in young people. There are usually systemic symptoms of infection such as headache, shivering and pyrexia before local discomfort begins to be felt in the area affected. The face, arm or leg are most often involved. The diagnosis has to be made from the appearance of the lesion as it is often difficult to isolate the streptococcus either from the involved area or from the blood.

Erysipelas may begin from a trivial local skin abrasion, an adjacent infected wound or sometimes from a distant source of infection. The lesion on the face is often associated with an upper respiratory tract infection. Benzyl penicillin remains the antibiotic of first choice, erythromycin is the best alternative in patients who are allergic to penicillin.

# Question 3.10

1. Name four abnormalities in this fundus.
2. List two other ocular abnormalities found in this condition.

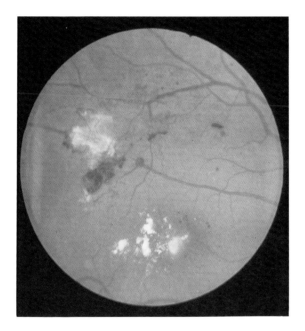

## Answer to question 3.10

1. Microaneurysms, hard exudates, dot and blot haemorrhages and new vessel formation.
2. Cataract, glaucoma and neovascularisation of the iris (rubeosis iridis).


This is diabetic retinopathy which is the main cause of blindness in the 20- to 65-year-old age group in the UK. Visual acuity should be carefully checked in every diabetic patient 3 months after their disease has become controlled. The fundi should be examined annually *always* after pupillary dilatation. The following patients should be referred to an ophthalmologist *before* visual acuity is impaired.

1. Those with neovascularisation anywhere in the retina.
2. Exudates near the fovea.
3. Evidence of ischaemia – i.e. cotton wool spots (micro-infarcts), venous irregularity and arterial sheathing.

# Question 3.11

This student took a job as an orderly in a large children's hospital after returning from extensive travels abroad.
1. What is this condition?
2. What treatment is indicated?
3. What further precautions should be taken in this case?

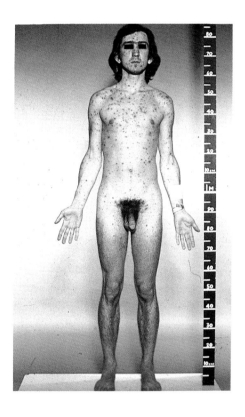

## Answer to question 3.11

1. Chickenpox.
2. None – unless signs of hepatitis or pneumonitis develop when intravenous anti-viral agents should be prescribed (e.g. acyclovir).
3. Strict isolation from and screening of susceptible immunocompromised patients.

In adults chicken pox may be a severe condition. The incubation period is 7–23 days and prodromal symptoms such as headache, backache and extreme malaise are common. There may be, as in smallpox, a transient pink rash before the vesicles erupt. Macules, papules, vesicles and scabs are all seen. They are superficial lesions, occurring in crops. The rash is centripetal and dense between the shoulder blades unlike that of smallpox which occurs centrifugally and particularly over the bony prominences.

Diagnosis is usually clinical but can be confirmed by paired sera taken ten days apart or by aspiration of vesicular fluid for culture.

Complications include secondary infection of the skin lesions, severe and sometimes fulminant pneumonitis, hepatitis, encephalitis, and venous thrombosis. Anti-viral treatment is advisable if any evidence of pneumonia or hepatitis exists and is mandatory for patients on long-term steroids or with lympho-proliferative disorders where the prognosis is particularly poor.

## Question 3.12

What would this appearance of the nails lead you to suspect?

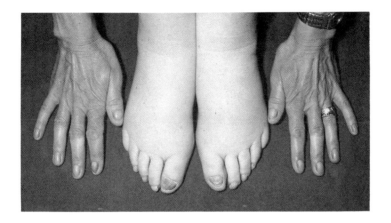

## Answer to question 3.12

Bronchiectasis. The yellow nail syndrome.

The yellow nail syndrome is a clinical association between discoloured yellow nails, hypoplastic lymphatics and bronchiectasis. The lymphatic hypoplasia results in chronic lymphoedema and pleural effusions. The mechanism of the bronchiectasis is unknown.

# Question 3.13

1. What is this skin lesion?
2. What features are characteristic on skin biopsy?

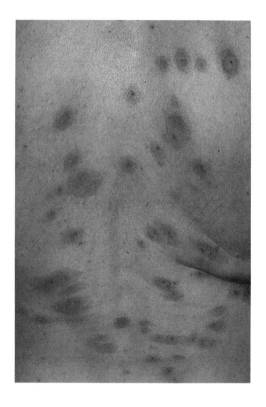

# Answer to question 3.13

1. Dermatitis herpetiformis.
2. Immunofluorescence of the skin would show both IgA and C3 attached to microfibrils in the sub-epidermis.


Dermatitis herpetiformis is a chronic itchy papulovesicular eruption usually on the extensor surfaces and symmetrically distributed. Its association with coeliac disease was first noted in 1966 and over 80% of patients with the disease have sub-total atrophy on intestinal biopsy. The xylose tolerance test is often abnormal. Many patients however do not have frank steatorrhea or symptoms. 77% of patients are of phenotype HLA-B8. The histological appearance of both IgA and C3 can be shown to be present in unaffected skin. Treatment is with a gluten-free diet and Dapsone if necessary.

# Question 3.14

1. What does this pathological specimen show?
2. List other pathological features with which this condition may be associated.

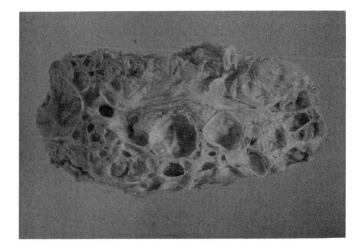

## Answer to question 3.14

**1.** Polycystic kidney
**2.** (a)  Cysts of liver, pancreas, spleen, uterus, ovary and
  lung.
  (b)  Berry aneurysm of the cerebral arteries.
  (c)  Secondary neoplasia in the kidney.

The adult form of polycystic disease is often inherited as an autosomal dominant and may present in the 3rd or 4th decade with renal impairment. Cysts of the liver and pancreas are found in up to 30% of patients. It may arise because of the failure of development of some nephric tubules but micropuncture studies have demonstrated that the cysts partake in both absorption and secretion.

Berry aneurysms occur in about 10% of patients and though neoplastic changes are rare they should be considered if a patient with polycystic kidneys develops weight loss, a PUO or persistent haematuria. The diagnosis is confirmed by ultrasound or intravenous urogram.

## Question 3.15

This man presented with a one year history of a gradually progressive skin rash with general symptoms of intense pruritus and weight loss.
1. What is the diagnosis?
2. How can this diagnosis be confirmed?

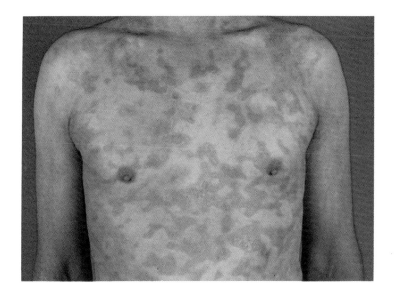

## Answer to question 3.15

**1.** Mycosis fungoides.
**2.** Skin biopsy.

Mycosis fungoides and the Sezary syndrome comprise the two main clinical syndromes of cutaneous lymphomas. They are characterised by infiltration of the skin by lymphocytes. The skin lesions have some features of chronic dermatitis and psoriasis. However, characteristically the plaques are raised and of inhomogeneous appearance with asymmetrical shape. The skin lesion, together with the systemic symptoms should raise the suspicion of a cutaneous lymphoma. The prognosis is frequently good initially with only minor symptoms for 10 or more years.

# Question 3.16

1. What is this lesion?
2. How may the diagnosis be confirmed?
3. What is the treatment?

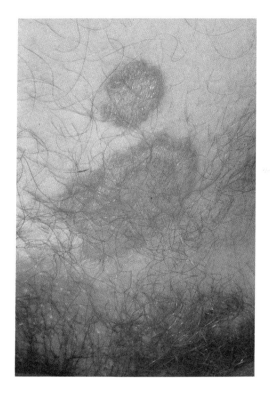

## Answer to question 3.16

1. Tinea cruris.
2. Direct microscopy of skin scales mounted in potassium hydroxide to demonstrate hyphae, and culture.
3. Usually topical treatment with clotrimazole.

Tinea cruris is a superficial fungal infection of the skin in the groin. The fungi causing this and related infections of other areas of skin, the nails and hair are known as the dermatophytes. Tinea cruris is most often caused by *Tricophyton rubrum* or *Epidermophyton floccosum*.

Tinea cruris is usually treated with clotrimazole, ecconazole or miconazole as topical therapy. Older therapies such as Whitfield's ointment (benzoic acid compound) may also be used. Griseofulvin may be given orally to patients with persistent or severe infections that have not responded to topical treatment.

# Question 3.17

1. What happened to the visual acuity of this eye?
2. What is the cause of this abnormality?
3. What should be examined in this patient?

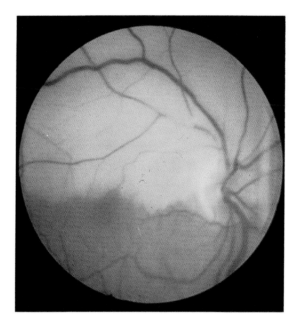

## Answer to question 3.17

1. There was an acute profound loss of vision in the area of retina supplied by this branch artery which is occluded.
2. An embolus which can be seen.
3. The carotid arteries and heart.

Retinal artery occlusion causes profound loss of vision in the affected area of the retina. The macula can sometimes be preserved by the presence of a cilioretinal vessel. Arterial occlusions are usually caused by emboli from either atherosclerotic plaques or calcified heart valves. However they may also be caused by atheroma and thrombosis in the vessel itself, hypertension, any form of vasculitis, fat emboli, SBE, diabetes or sickle cell disease.

## Question 3.18

Blood was taken from this patient who was admitted semi-conscious and the casualty officer noticed this appearance of the blood sample which had stood for a few minutes prior to collection.

What would be your explanation?

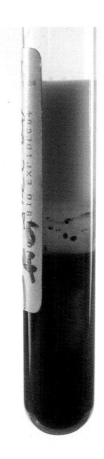

## Answer to question 3.18

Acute pancreatitis.

Separation of the blood in this way may be seen in patients with acute pancreatitis. Hypertriglyceridaemia occurs in 15–20% and may antedate the acute event. Often the serum amylase is low in these patients even though serum lipase activity is high suggesting that an anti-amylase may be present in the serum. Other factors which will contribute to the cell/plasma separation are haemoconcentration, hypocalcaemia, leucocytosis, hypoalbuminaemia and hyperbilirubinaemia.

# Question 3.19

1. What is this condition?
2. How should the diagnosis be confirmed?
3. What is the prognosis?

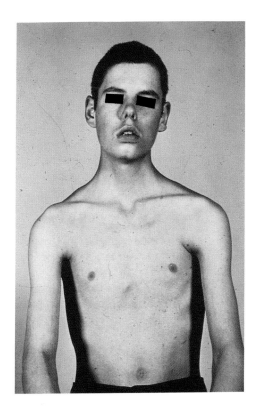

# Answer to question 3.19

**1.** Facioscapulohumeral muscular dystrophy.
**2.** Electromyography.
**3.** A normal life expectancy.

This degenerative myopathy is inherited as an autosomal dominant trait. It is usually first recognised in adolescence and unlike the Duchenne type of dystrophy, muscular enlargement is uncommon. Facial involvement with pouting lips and difficulty closing the eyes is characteristic and is accompanied by weakness in the shoulder girdle muscles with 'winging' of the scapulae and pectoral wasting. The condition usually runs a benign and prolonged course with cessation of the disease process after certain groups of muscles have been affected. However, progression to involve the lower extremities (characteristically the anterior tibial muscles with associated foot drop) and lumbar spine with muscular contractures and spinal deformity may occur. The myocardium is not affected and intelligence is normal.

Electromyography confirms the appearances of any myopathy: namely, absent spontaneous activity in the relaxed resting muscle with characteristic appearances on voluntary movement. If clinical appearances are unusual EMG helps to distinguish between muscular dystrophy and spinal neuropathic disorders. Muscle biopsy with histochemical analysis may be needed to distinguish between primary myopathic changes and those secondary to denervation from spinal disease.

# Question 3.20

The patient, aged 43, was referred by his GP because of occasional attacks of loose stool, 3–4 times a day, occurring for a few days every few months over the last six years. There was blood and mucus on one occasion. Sigmoidoscopy showed a granular mucosa and barium enema was normal.

What does this specimen of stool show?

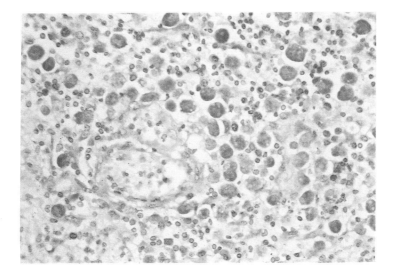

## Answer to question 3.20

The cysts of *Entamoeba histolytica*.


*E. Histolytica* is one of the seven species of amoebae found in man and the only one to cause disease. It is endemic worldwide and the majority of patients are asymptomatic carriers, with an occasional attack of loose stool. More severe amoebic dysentery is seen in those who are pregnant or on steroids when ulcers are seen in the colon and trophozoites are excreted in the stool. Systemic invasion with hepatic abscess formation is becoming rarer. The differential diagnosis is between campylobacter, shigella, salmonella, ulcerative colitis or diverticular disease and these tend to produce neutrophils in the stool which are not found in amoebic infestation. Serology may be negative in those in whom tissue invasion has not occured and remains positive in patients who have had systemic invasion for many months or years.

# Paper 4

# Question 4.1

1. What does this autopsy specimen show?
2. If you were the pathologist for what other finding would you look?

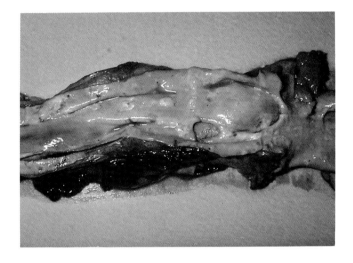

## Answer to question 4.1

**1.** Dissection of the aorta.
**2.** Left ventricular hypertrophy.

The two commonest sites for aortic dissection are just above the aortic valve and just beyond the origin of the left subclavian artery. Idiopathic cystic medionecrosis or a similar condition seen in Marfans syndrome may be the first lesion. It has been suggested that the initial blood leak may be from the vasa vasorum and then connection is established between the rupture and the aortic lumen. Further tearing will depend on the angular shearing forces and the wavelength of the harmonics which go to make up the pressure pulse transmitted by cardiac systole. The shorter the tear and the greater the length of the pulse wave the less likely it is to extend. Most commonly aortic dissection occurs in the elderly with undiagnosed systemic hypertension (left ventricular wall thickness greater than 15 mm). Clinically there is chest pain followed by loss of pulses, collapse, pericardial tamponade or aortic incompetence. The dissection may rupture back into the aorta to produce a double-barrelled aorta.

Diagnosis is by arteriography although some information may be obtained from ultrasound in experienced hands. The priority is to lower blood pressure provided the cardiac output is adequate and ask for surgical advice.

# Question 4.2

1. What is the diagnosis?
2. What is the most common complication?

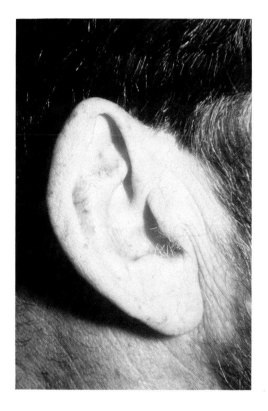

## Answer to question 4.2

1. Hereditary haemorrhagic telangiectasia (Osler-Rendu-Weber syndrome).
2. Iron deficiency anaemia due to gastrointestinal haemorrhage.

This condition is inherited as autosomal dominant and may not become clinically apparent until adult life. Multiple telangiectases are found in the skin and mucous membranes and are raised, red lesions 2–3 mm in diameter which blanch on pressure. Nose bleeds and chronic or rarely acute gastrointestinal haemorrhage from bowel lesions may lead to anaemia. Treatment is conservative with pressure to accessible bleeding points but surgical intervention may be necessary for severe gastrointestinal bleeds.

# Question 4.3

1. What is the diagnosis?
2. Why is this picture uncharacteristic of this condition?
3. What is the cause?

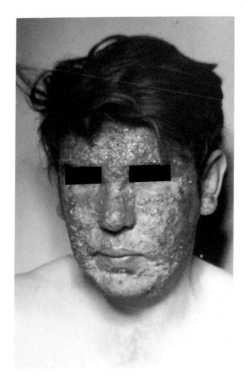

## Answer to question 4.3

1. Impetigo.
2. It is mainly found in children rather than adults.
3. Either *Staphylococcus aureus* or group A streptococcus or both.

This condition is found commonly in children in poor socioeconomic conditions. It is a localised infection of the superficial layers of the skin. It is frequently found on skin already damaged by scabies, insect bites or minor trauma. Most cases are caused by *Staph. aureus*, although group A streptococci can be found. Sometimes both organisms are cultured from the lesions. If *Staph. aureus* is found a penicillinase resistant antibiotic such as flucloxacillin should be employed and benzyl penicillin used for streptococcal infections.

## Question 4.4

This lesion caused refractory pruritus.
1. What is this condition?
2. Name three drugs with which it may be associated.

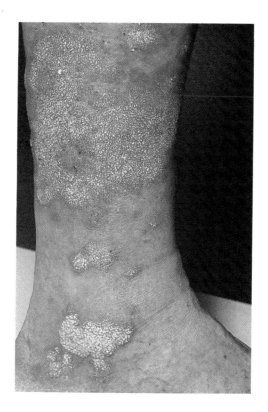

## Answer to question 4.4

1. Lichen planus.
2. Gold, penicillamine, organic arsenicals, antituberculous therapy, phenothiazines and methyldopa.

The lesions are characteristically violaceous papules symmetrically distributed on the flexor surfaces of the wrists and legs. They may also be found on the trunk, glans penis and on the oral and vaginal mucosa.

The cause of primary lichen planus is unknown; an immunological basis is probable. The drugs listed above, graft-versus-host disease and systemic lupus erythematosis may give a similar clinical and histological appearance.

## Question 4.5

This patient is a club manager.
1. What two abnormalities are shown?
2. What is this condition?
3. What investigations would help to confirm the diagnosis?

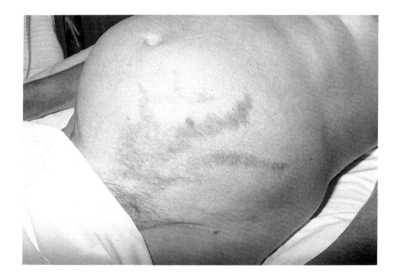

## Answer to question 4.5

**1.** Ascites, striae.
**2.** Pseudo-Cushing's syndrome induced by alcohol abuse.
**3.** 24-hour urinary cortisol and liver biopsy.


Alcoholic patients may exhibit many of the features of Cushing's syndrome including moon facies, plethora, thin skin and striae. High plasma cortisol levels are usually found in pseudo-Cushing's syndrome induced by alcohol and they may not supress with dexamethasone. The biochemical features return to normal after abstention from alcohol for a few weeks and this may be the only way to differentiate it from true Cushing's syndrome.

# Question 4.6

1. What is the diagnosis?
2. What other features may be present?

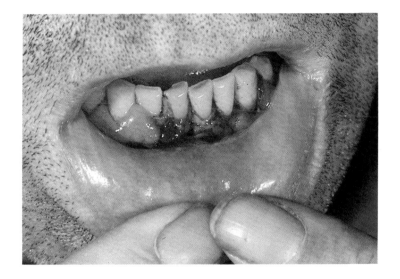

## Answer to question 4.6

1. Scurvy.
2. Cork-screw hairs, spontaneous ecchymoses, anaemia and periostitis.


Vitamin C deficiency prevents the normal hydroxylation of proto-collagen to collagen and the main manifestation is poor wound healing and cutaneous changes with blood vessel dilatation and haemorrhage giving purpuric macules which coalesce, especially in the legs. Gum changes are also prominent especially in those with gingivitis and dental caries. They are said not to occur in edentulous patients.

# Question 4.7

This patient was from West Africa. He was suffering from severe pain in his right hip. On examination he was also found to have an abnormal fundus.
1. What are these retinal changes due to?
2. What was the cause of the pain his hip?
3. What is the most likely diagnosis?

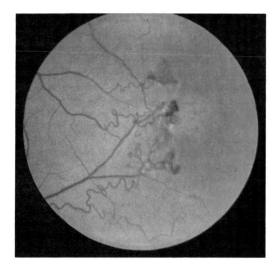

## Answer to question 4.7

1. Capillary occlusion due to sickled red blood cells resulting in new vessel formation.
2. Aseptic necrosis of the femoral head.
3. Haemoglobin SC disease.

The changes seen in this fundus may be seen in sickle cell disease but are more common in haemoglobin SC disease. This is probably due to the higher haemoglobin found in patients with haemoglobin SC disease as well as the effects of sickling and increased red cell fragility caused by haemoglobin C. The disorder results in retinitis proliferans, retinal detachment and sometimes permanent blindness.

# Question 4.8

1. What is this lesion?
2. What other cutaneous lesions may be present?
3. What two blood tests should be used to confirm the diagnosis?

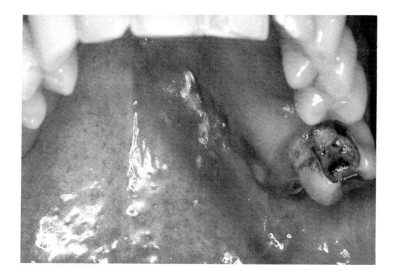

## Answer to question 4.8

**1.** Snail track ulcer of secondary syphilis.
**2.** (a)  Macular (sometimes papular) coppery rash.
    (b)  Condylomata lata.
**3.** Serological tests of VDRL, and TPHA/FTA.

Syphilis has an incubation period of 9–90 days. Secondary syphilis may be bypassed but classically develops six weeks after the primary chancre disappears. Snail track ulcers are painless greyish erosions forming circles and arches on the mucous membranes of the mouth and are highly infectious. Classically a coppery coloured rash is found upon the trunk and proximal limbs but most characteristically on the palms, soles and face. It is painless, non-irritant and symmetrical. Condyloma lata are papules enlarging into pink or grey discs found in warm moist areas such as the perineum, perianal region, axilla and under the breasts. Other features of the condition include: (a) mild constitutional disturbance with malaise and lymphadenopathy; (b) alopecia, laryngitis, hepatitis with elevated alkaline phosphatase and rarely a nephrotic syndrome; (c) periostitis and uveitis may be present. All these lesions may disappear although 20–25% of patients left untreated develop relapsing secondary syphilis over the next 2–4 years.

Serological tests include those using non-specific reagin antibodies (IgG, IgM) and specific anti-treponaemal antibodies. The venereal disease research laboratory test (VDRL) is a non-specific test but is quantitative and the titres reflect activity. This may be the only evidence of reinfection in a patient with previously treated syphilis in whom the VDRL was previously negative or only weakly positive. False positive VDRL is usually of low titre (1:8 or less) and a sharp rise of titre of 4-fold or higher is good evidence of active infection even with negative clinical signs. The fluorescent treponaemal antibody test (FTA-ABS) is the most specific and sensitive test known for syphilis. It does not assess activity and stays positive long after therapy. The treponaemal haemagglutination test (TPHA) is simpler but less specific than the FTA and with the VDRL is the best combination of tests for routine use.

# Question 4.9

This patient complained of chronic constipation and intermittent abdominal pain of two years' duration. Barium enema showed incomplete emptying and streaks of gas within the bowel wall and mesentery.
1. What is the diagnosis?
2. What complication is indicated by the barium enema?
3. What immunological abnormality may be present?

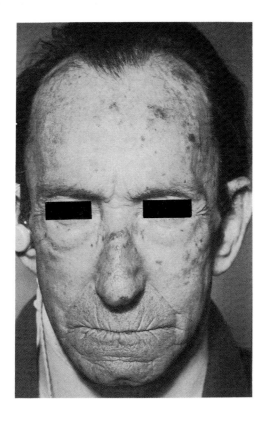

# Answer to question 4.9

1. Scleroderma (progressive systemic sclerosis).
2. Pneumatosis cystoides intestinalis.
3. Positive anti-nuclear antigen is present in 20–80% of patients mainly of the speckled or nucleolar pattern. An increased incidence of HLA A1, B8 and DR3 has been reported.

Scleroderma is a generalised disease secondary to degeneration of collagen affecting the skin and small vessels with intimal thickening and vessel obliteration. The patients may present with Raynaud's phenomenon (90%), a polyarthritis (25%), gastrointestinal, renal, cardiac or lung involvement. In the gastrointestinal tract 50% of patients are affected, but only half of these are symptomatic with oesophageal dilatation, hiatus hernia, oesophageal reflux and stricture formation. Malabsorption may occur and colonic involvement may result in diarrhoea or constipation. The streaks of gas seen on X-ray mentioned here are due to pneumatosis cystoides intestinalis with which scleroderma is associated.

Cutaneous lesions (as shown here) may begin as subtle oedema, followed by skin tightening and contraction. This usually occurs in the distal tips of the fingers but may spread up to the forearms. Involvement of the face feet and legs may also occur. Calcification of the finger tips, Raynaud's phenomenon, scleroderma and telangiectasia form the CRST variant.

## Question 4.10

This skin eruption has its highest incidence in the spring and autumn.
1. What is the diagnosis?
2. What is the differential diagnosis?
3. What is the treatment?

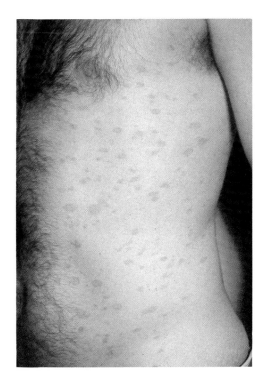

## Answer to question 4.10

1. Pityriasis rosacea.
2. Secondary syphilis is the most important; others include tinea corporis, tinea versicolor, drug eruptions and psoriasis.
3. No specific treatment, the lesion resolves spontaneously.

Pityriasis rosacea is a self-limiting skin eruption which is probably due to a virus. It occurs most commonly in the spring and autumn. A characteristic 'herald' patch is usually present 5–10 days before the main lesions appear. The lesions are found mainly on the trunk and proximal parts of the limbs, they are oval with their long axes lying along the line markings of the skin. There is seldom any systemic disturbance but a mild pyrexia and lymphadenopathy may occur occasionally. Intense pruritus may be troublesome. The condition is self-limiting, lasting for 3–6 weeks.

# Question 4.11

This patient presented with progressively increasing shortness of breath.
1. What is the diagnosis?
2. What confirmatory tests would you perform?

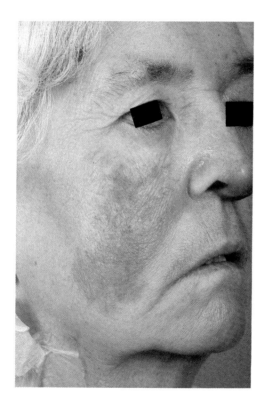

# Answer to question 4.11

1. Sarcoidosis.
2. Kveim test, transfer factor for carbon monoxide, transbronchial lung biopsy.

9% of patients with sarcoid may have skin lesions other than erythema nodosum (lupus pernio, transient maculopapular eruptions, leucoderma and keloid-like reactions at scars). Lupus pernio is a persistent violaceous lesion with a predeliction for the nose and is associated with sarcoid of the upper respiratory tract. The Kveim test is positive in 80% of all patients with sarcoid but suffers from the disadvantage that biopsy is performed six weeks after the insertion of the antigen. Some physicians would perform a bronchoscopy and biopsy which reveals granulomata compatible with sarcoid and the transfer factor for carbon monoxide will be reduced if interstitial pulmonary involvement has occurred.

## Question 4.13

This woman's chest X-ray is clear.
1. What is this lesion?
2. What is the underlying diagnosis?
3. How should this diagnosis be confirmed?

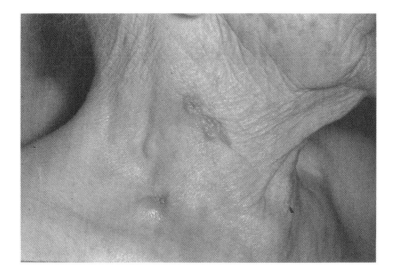

## Answer to question 4.13

1. Cervical lymphadenitis with chronically discharging sinus.
2. Lymph node tuberculosis.
3. Lymph node biopsy and histological examination.

Lymph node tuberculosis (TB) in the UK is predominantely a disease of African and Asian imigrants (75% of all cases). Lymphadenitis occurs predominantely in the cervical region and forms more than half of the non-respiratory TB occurring in this ethnic group. At the beginning of the 20th century the disease in Europe was frequently due to the bovine organism, but now mycobacterium tuberculosis is most commonly isolated. In African and Asian imigrants to the UK cervical lymphadenitis is often associated with TB in the lungs or elsewhere but this is not invariably the case. Lymph node swelling may progress to the formation of abcesses and chronically discharging sinuses which leave unsightly scars. Bacterial confirmation is hindered by the fact that there is a low isolation rate (60%) on culture from biopsy. Consequently histological examination following node biopsy is the diagnostic method of choice. During chemotherapy the nodes may enlarge, shrink or ulcerate further with development of new sinuses. Surgical drainage may be necessary, although the final outcome is excellent, providing chemotherapy is continuous.

## Question 4.14

Of what cell types might this tumour be composed?

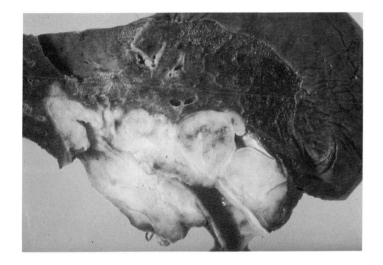

## Answer to question 4.14

1. Squamous cell
2. Oat cell (small cell)
3. Adenocarcinoma
4. Large cell undifferentiated

Squamous cell carcinoma of the bronchus is the commonest histological type (35%), followed by small cell (oat cell) tumours (24%) thought to be derived from neurosecretory (APUD) cells which may explain the high incidence (6–8%) of endocrine syndromes with this tumour. Adenocarcinoma (21%) tend to occur peripherally, is not associated with smoking and is more common in women. The large cell undifferentiated (19%) or polygonal cell tumours account for the rest. It has been suggested that the incidence of squamous and oat cell carcinomas is increasing. Despite the advent of precise histology and accurate staging the 5-year survival remains at only 6–8%.

# Question 4.15

1. What three abnormalities are present on this blood film?
2. What procedure has been carried out on this patient?

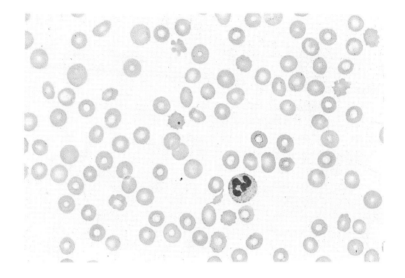

## Answer to question 4.15

1. (a) Howell-Jolly bodies.
   (b) Target cells.
   (c) Irregularly contracted or crenated red cells.
2. Splenectomy.

These are the haematological changes following splenectomy. The proportion of the various cell types seen depends upon the presence or abscence of underlying dyserythropoiesis. In patients with haemolytic anaemias, thallassaemia and sideroblastic anaemias a major portion of the red cells may contain siderotic granules. The number of Howell Jolly bodies is variable and most marked when there is underlying dyserythropoiesis.

This blood picture may also be seen in patients with hyposplenism. The causes of this include coeliac disease, dermatitis herpetiformis, ulcerative colitis, sickle cell anamia, essential thrombocythaemia and Fanconi's syndrome.

# Question 4.16

1. Name two abnormal features.
2. Is there any connection between these features?
3. Name two complications of the skin lesion.

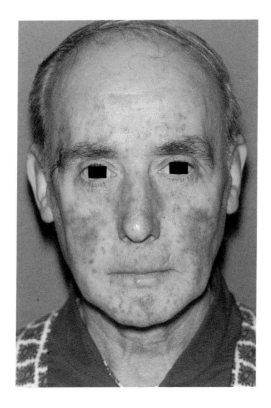

## Answer to question 4.16

1. Acne rosacea, temporal artery biopsy.
2. No.
3. Rhinophyma, blepharitis, keratitis.


Acne rosacea is confined to the 'flush' areas of the forehead, nose, cheeks and chin and results from overactivity of sebaceous glands induced by hyperaemia. Lesions rarely appear on the neck and upper arms. Unlike acne vulgaris there is no duct blockage and comedones are not formed, but inflammation around the hypertrophied gland occurs.

Facial flushing underlies this process and any reason for chronic flushing may result in these lesions.

Hypertrophy of the sebaceous glands can occur to such an extent on the nose that it becomes bulbous or lobulated – a condition known as rhinophyma. Some sufferers of acne rosacea show symptoms of dermatitis such as scruffy scalp and blepharitis. Conjunctivitis is associated with the latter. Rarely a severe superficial keratitis with photophobia, lacrimation and visual disturbance results.

Treatment consists of avoidance of those things that lead to flushing, especially alcohol. Topical preparations and low dose tetracycline may be effective. The temporal artery biopsy shown in this patient is incidental.

# Question 4.17

1. What does this patient show?
2. What would be your presumptive diagnosis?

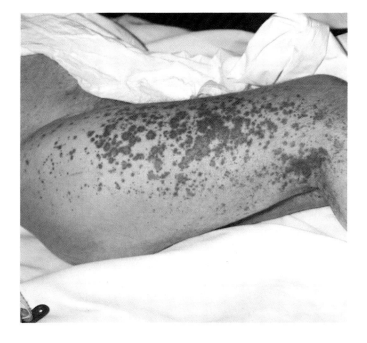

## Answer to question 4.17

**1.** Purpura.
**2.** Septicaemia.

Septic shock may be clinically obvious but, as in this patient, no source of infection was apparent. The endotoxin causes endothelial cell damage and an abrupt thrombocytopenia and granulocytopenia. These damaged cells cause release of blood coagulation factors, complement activation products and fibrin is laid down in many tissues. Deficiency of clotting factors due to consumption is a feature of disseminated intravascular coagulation (DIC).

Adrenal haemorrhage with septicaemia (Waterhouse-Friderichsen syndrome) may produce a superadded acute adrenal crisis.

# Question 4.18

1. What three physical signs are evident?
2. What is the diagnosis?
3. What single test would confirm your suspicions?

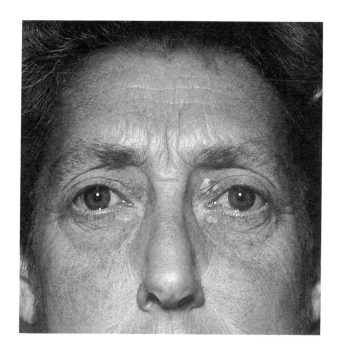

## Answer to question 4.18

1. Jaundice, skin pigmentation and xanthelasmata.
2. Primary biliary cirrhosis.
3. Mitochondrial antibody in serum.

Primary biliary cirrhosis is most commonly found in middle-aged females (90% of cases). They usually present with pruritus (50%), dark urine and pale stools or steathorroea with malabsorption due to the lack of intestinal bile acids. A raised IgM is found in 80% but the most consistent finding is the presence of mitochondrial antibodies in 95%. The lack of excretion of bile acids and cholesterol results in hypercholesterolaemia with xanthelasmata and tendon xanthomata. The skin pigmentation is due to increased melanin in the basal layer in light exposed areas.

## Question 4.19

This patient had successful treatment for severe rheumatoid arthritis but developed some disturbance of vision.
1. What was the cause of the visual disturbance?
2. What changes may be found in the eye in this situation?

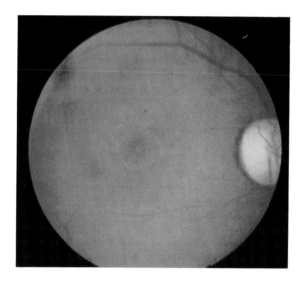

## Answer to question 4.19

**1.** Chloroquine.
**2.** Keratopathy and retinopathy – in particular, macular degeneration.

Chloroquine retinopathy does not usually occur before a total dose of 100 g has been given and the drug used for over a year. Chloroquine keratopathy is the deposition of chloroquine crystals in the cornea. They disappear, leaving no damage, if the drug is stopped and sometimes even if the drug is continued. Chloroquine retinopathy however is not reversible. It is characterised by a ring of depigmentation surrounding the macula with a zone of pigmentation surrounding this – giving the classical 'bull's eye' appearance. Other changes that may be found are attenuation of the arterioles and a waxy appearance of the optic disc. Patients being given long-term chloroquine should be told to report any disturbance of vision immediately and be seen regularly by an ophthalmologist.

## Question 4.20

1. What is the cause of this lesion?
2. How would you establish the diagnosis?
3. Is there any effective treatment?

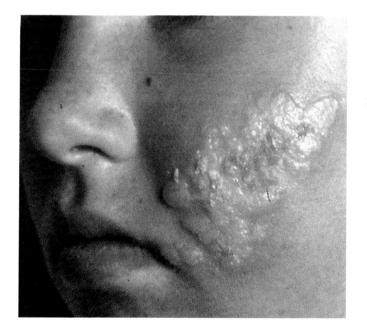

## Answer to question 4.20

1. Lesion caused by herpes simplex type I.
2. Swabs should be taken and sent to the laboratory in Hanks's transport medium. Sera may be taken when the patient is first seen and ten days later.
3. Idoxuridine, cytarabine, vidarabine and acyclovir have all been shown to be effective.

Most herpes simplex infections are caused by the type I virus. The type II virus usually causes genital herpes and disease in the newborn. The mouth and lips are the usual site of the primary infection. It is often trivial in children but many people are not infected in childhood. Primary infections in adolescents and adults are often more severe as in this case. If the appropriate swabs are taken the virus is easily cultured in the laboratory and rising titres of antibody are found in the serum. Medical and dental personnel are sometimes infected on the hands (the herpetic whitlow) from patients actively secreting the virus particularly from the mouth and lips. For relatively trivial cutaneous lesions, a topical application of a 35% solution of idoxuridine in dimelthyl-sulphoxide is often used. For more severe infections acyclovir has become the treatment of choice. However, it should not be used indiscriminantly as viruses resistant to acyclovir have been reported.

# Paper 5

# Question 5.1

1. What is this condition?
2. What is it caused by?
3. Why is it now less common than previously?

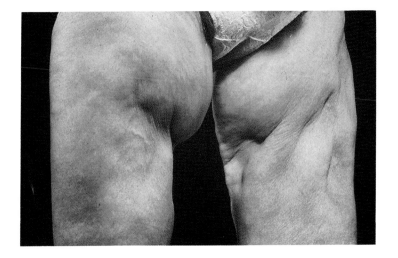

## Answer to question 5.1

1. Lipoatrophy.
2. It is the loss of subcutaneous fat at the site of insulin injection.
3. It is less common now highly purified insulins are being used.

The lipodystrophies (lipoatrophy/lipohypertrophy) are the second most common complication of insulin therapy; hypoglycaemia being the commonest. Lipoatrophy is very uncommon in patients using the purified insulins. The best treatment for the problem is to inject a purified insulin into the centre and margins of the atrophic area. The abnormal areas gradually improve when this technique is used. Lipohypertrophy is due to the repeated injection of insulin into one area. Avoidance of this site of injection allows the hypertrophic area to resolve.

# Question 5.2

This patient presented with acute shortness of breath.
**1.** What operation might he have had?
**2.** List one further complication of this condition.

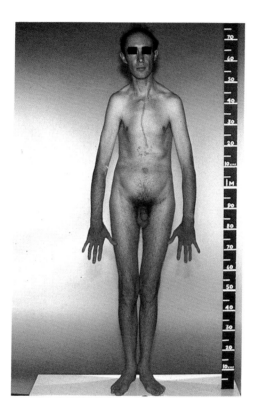

# Answer to question 5.2

1. Aortic or mitral valve replacement, repair of aortic dissection or coarctation.
2. Dislocation of the lens in the eye.

Marfan syndrome is a disorder of connective tissue inherited as an autosomal dominant trait. It results in skeletal, cardiovascular and ocular abnormalities.

The skeletal abnormalities include long tubular bones, arachnodactyly, arm span exceeds height, pectus excavation or carinatum and hyperextensible joints.

In the cardiovascular system the abnormality of the aortic media leads to weakness of the wall resulting in aortic dilatation and possible dissection. Mitral incompetence, subacute bacterial endocarditis and coarctation of the aorta are also found.

The ocular changes are most commonly dislocation of the lens and high grade myopia with retinal detachment.

# Question 5.3

What does this lung show?

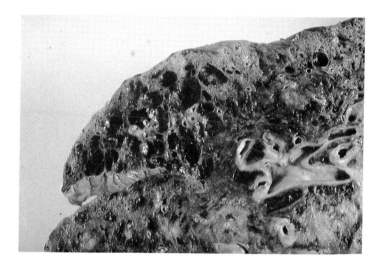

## Answer to question 5.3

Emphysema.

Emphysema is a pathological definition of destruction and dilatation of the air spaces distal to the respiratory bronchiole and is difficult to recognise clinically unless severe. Loss of lung elastic recoil is pathognomonic but unhelpful in a clinical setting. It is a feature of advancing age although the major causative factor is smoking which also produces the airflow limitation of chronic bronchitis – a disease from which emphysema can rarely be totally separated.

In a non-smoker the presence of emphysema at an early age should suggest deficiency of alpha-l-antitrypsin (homozygous genotype ZZ) which has an incidence of 1 in 3000. This has lead to the proposal that emphysema represents an auto-destruction of the lung parenchyma by either deficiency of a protective enzyme or a disturbance in the balance between proteases and anti-proteases.

# Question 5.4

1. What is the abnormality in this picture?
2. What is the most common cause of this abnormality?
3. Name one other cause.

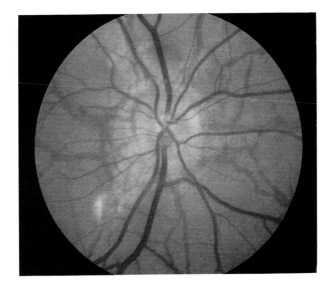

## Answer to question 5.4

1. Angioid streaks.
2. Pseudoxanthoma elasticum.
3. Sickle cell anaemia.

Angioid streaks were originally thought to be due to abnormal vessels but they are, in fact, linear cracks in an abnormal Bruch's membrane and are located behind the normal retinal vasculature. Disciform degeneration of the macula is a common occurrence which leads to severe loss of vision. They occur most commonly in pseudoxanthoma elasticum and Ehlers-Danlos syndrome but may also be seen in sickle cell anaemia, Paget's disease and rarely acromegaly, hypercalcaemia and lead poisoning.

# Question 5.5

1. What is the diagnosis?
2. Name two possible causes.
3. Name three other causes of short stature.

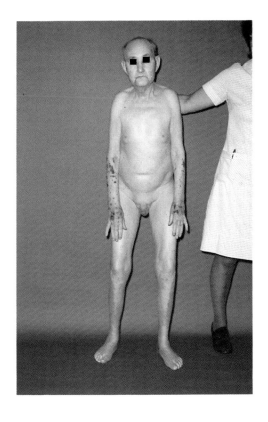

## Answer to question 5.5

1. Panhypopituitarism.
2. Congenital or a pituitary tumour.

   In the adult panhypopituitarism may occur (but with normal stature) due to a pituitary tumour (primary or secondary); after pituitary surgery; with infectious disease (e.g. tuberculosis); granulomatous disease (e.g. sarcoidosis); vascular disease (e.g. postpartum) or post-traumatic.
3. Constitutional delay in growth, familial short stature, hypothyroidism, coeliac disease, achondroplasia and precocious puberty.

This patient has congenital panhypopituitarism. This is usually transmitted by autosomal recessive inheritance but occasionally dominant or X-linked inheritance may occur. The growth *in utero* is not retarded in this condition, which can help to separate it from congenital hypothyroidism in which fetal growth is impaired. The condition is not usually diagnosed until the child is approaching school age when retarded growth becomes more noticeable. However, recognition of a micropenis is an early diagnostic clue. As shown above there are many causes of hypopituitarism; the commonest cause is now a pituitary tumour. A prolactin secreting tumour is the most likely in adults and a craniopharyngioma in children. The most common causes of short stature are constitutional delay in growth and familial short stature with the other causes being much rarer. Therefore, a very careful clinical assessment including percentile chart measurements should be carried out before more extensive investigations are undertaken.

## Question 5.6

This patient originally presented with shortness of breath on exertion and ankle oedema.
1. What was the diagnosis?
2. What is the particular feature shown here?

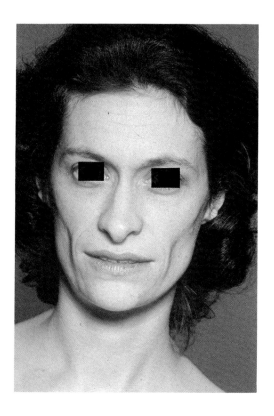

## Answer to question 5.6

1. Nephrotic syndrome secondary to mesangiocapillary glomerulo-nephritis.
2. Facial lipodystrophy.

Mesangiocapillary glomerulonephritis (MCGN) mainly affects adolescents and young adults and usually presents with haematuria, proteinuria or frank nephrotic syndrome. 50% of patients reach end-stage renal failure within seven years. Two pathological types are described whereby glomerular mesangial cells proliferate either subendothelially (type 1) or within the capillary basement membrane (type 2). Abnormalities of the complement system involving intermittment or prolonged reduction in C3 and the detection of C3 nephritic factor are described. Partial lipodystrophy, the loss of subcutaneous fat in various parts of the body including the face, upper limbs and trunk, is a rare accompaniment to this condition and is usually associated with type 2 MCGN.

# Question 5.7

What test would you do to confirm the diagnosis?

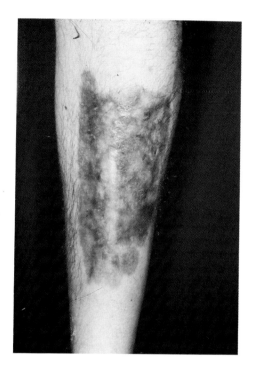

## Answer to question 5.7

Glucose tolerance test.

Necrobiosis lipoidica diabeticorum may be the first presenting sign of diabetes mellitus. It occurs three times more commonly in women than men and begins as a nodule and eventually results in an indolent shallow ulcer. Histology reveals dermal collagen containing fat-laden cells and capillaries infiltrated by PAS positive material. The latter feature is also seen in the micro-angiopathy of diabetes. Some patients have a normal blood sugar but their glucose tolerance test is abnormal. Normalisation of blood glucose is thought to have little effect on their resolution and most resolve spontaneously over two or three years.

# Question 5.8

1. Of what is the appearance of this blood film suggestive?
2. List three underlying causes.

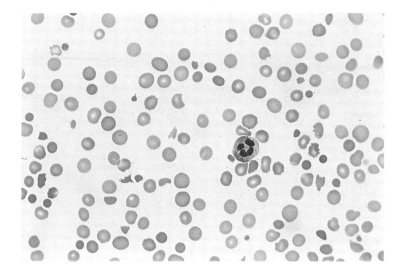

## Answer to question 5.8

1. Microangiopathic haemolytic anaemia (MAHA). This diagnosis is made largely on the morphological appearance of the red cells in the film which show marked fragmentation and the presence of many microspherocytes. Numerous oddly shaped red cells are seen including 'helmet cells'. The Coombs' test is normally negative.
2. MAHA is due to mechanical destruction of red cells as a result of a variety of pathological changes in small blood vessels. The condition has been described in association with a wide variety of systemic disorders which include malignant hypertension, disseminated carcinomatosis, the connective tissue diseases, septicaemia, and acute glomerulonephritis.

# Question 5.9

This patient presented with abdominal pain and vomiting.
1. What is the cause of the symptoms?
2. What is unusual about the patient in this photograph?
3. If a skin biopsy is taken what is found on immunofluorescence?

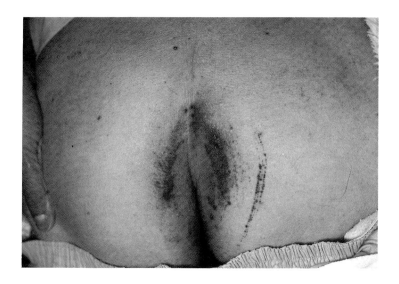

## Answer to question 5.9

1. Intussusception of the small intestine.
2. This condition is much more common in children than in adults.
3. IgA is found deposited in the walls of involved vessels.

This patient has Henoch-Schönlein purpura. This condition is a self-limiting disorder in which a small vessel vasculitis is found. It is characterised by purpura, arthritis and gastrointestinal and renal lesions. The pathogenesis is unknown. 90% of cases are preceded by an upper respiratory tract infection. β-haemolytic streptococci are isolated in one third of these. Some drugs, such as sulphonamides and pencillins have been implicated as initiating agents. Vasculitis in the small vessels of the bowel wall causes inflammation and oedema, often associated with abdominal pain and bleeding. Some gastrointestinal involvement occurs in about 60% of cases and may be complicated by intussusception, infarction or perforation. Renal involvement is characterised by a focal glomerulonephritis. IgA, $C_3$ and properdin may be found by immunofluorescence in the renal biopsy. Children and adolescents are most commonly affected with boys outnumbering girls by 2:1.

# Question 5.10

This patient presented with colicky abdominal pain.
1. What is the lesion in the picture?
2. What caused the abdominal pain?
3. Would a plain abdominal X-ray help in this situation?

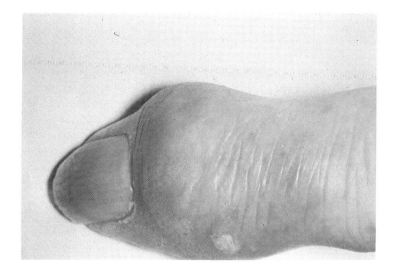

## Answer to question 5.10

1. A gouty tophus.
2. Renal colic due to uric acid urolithiasis.
3. No – because pure uric acid renal calculi are radiolucent.

The majority of patients with hyperuricaemia never develop arthritis due to gout. Therefore, arthritis associated with hyperuricaemia is not diagnostic of gout. The diagnosis can be confirmed by either a typical history, with recurrent acute mono-articular arthritis associated with hyperuricaemia, or the finding of gouty tophi, or the presence of monosodium urate crystals in the synovial fluid from an inflamed joint.

The incidence of urolithiasis is 1000 times greater in patients with gout than in the general population. Free uric acid precipitates out as crystals in an acidic urine where they may form radiolucent calculi.

Other medical conditions associated with hyperuricaemia and gout are the myeloproliferative disorders, psoriasis, myxoedema, hypo- and hyperparathyroidism, obesity, hypertension, ischaemic heart disease and chronic renal failure.

# Question 5.11

1. What is the most likely diagnosis?
2. List four differential diagnoses.
3. List three symptoms and three signs that are clinically helpful.

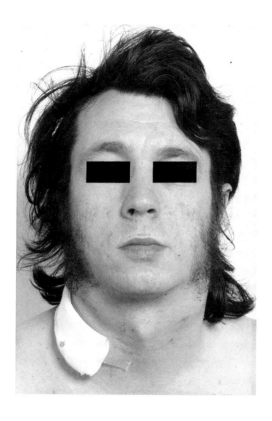

## Answer to question 5.11

1. Hodgkin's disease.
2. Infectious mononucleosis, toxoplasmosis, cytomegalovirus infection, lymphatic leukaemia, non-Hodgkin's lymphoma, sarcoidosis, tuberculosis or secondary carcinoma.
3. Unexplained weight loss, fever and night sweats. Distribution of lymphadenopathy, splenomegaly and evidence of extralymphatic organ involvement.


Lymphadenopathy is the first abnormality noticed by the majority of patients with Hodgkin's disease which was the diagnosis in this young man. The cell type, symptoms and signs listed above are important as they help to stage the disease which determines the treatment that the patient is given.

## Question 5.12

This is the fundus of a 9-year-old child.
1. Name two abnormal physical signs seen in this picture.
2. What is this condition?

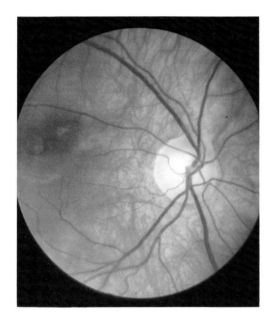

## Answer to question 5.12

**1.** Pigmentary macular degeneration, retinal degeneration, optic atrophy.

**2.** Subacute sclerosing panencephalitis (SSPE).

This condition follows 5–10 years after a normal measles infection. It is due to persistence of the virus leading to a slowly progressive neurological disease. There is a gradual deterioration in personality and intellect, followed by seizures, pyramidal and extrapyramidal signs and finally decerebrate rigidity. In the eye optic neuritis and pigmentary macular degeneration are found followed by retinal necrosis and optic atrophy.

The electro-encephalogram is characteristic; there are high titres of antibody to the virus in both the blood and CSF and the virus may be isolated from the brain. The incidence of SSPE following a normal measles infection is ten times greater than that following vaccination. The prognosis is poor.

## Question 5.13

1. What two abnormal physical signs are present?
2. Name two differential diagnoses for these lesions.
3. What single test would help to determine the site of the lesion?

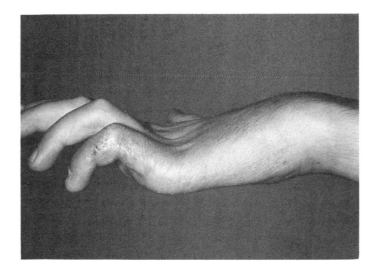

## Answer to question 5.13

1. Claw hand and skin damage associated with sensory impairment.
2. Ulnar nerve palsy and eighth cervical root lesion.
3. Nerve conduction studies.

This picture demonstrates the classical features of an ulnar nerve ($C_7$, $C_8$ and $T_1$) or eighth cervical root lesion. Branches of the ulnar nerve to flexor carpi ulnaris and the medial part of flexor digitorum profundus arise in the upper arm. However, these branches travel with the main nerve trunk in the ulnar groove at the elbow. Therefore, lesions at the elbow affecting the main trunk usually damage these branches resulting in weakness of flexion of the 4th and 5th fingers. In the forearm the dorsal branch arises which supplies the skin over part of the dorsum of the hand and the dorsum of the medial one and a half fingers. Damage to the three branches mentioned distinguishes lesions at the elbow from those of the wrist.

The main nerve passes into the hand superficial to the flexor retinaculum. It first supplies a superficial sensory branch to the medial part of the palm and medial one and a half fingers and then motor branches to the hypothenar muscles, all the interossei, the third and fourth lumbricals, the adductor pollicis and part of the flexor pollicis brevis. If damage occurs distal to the superficial sensory branch there is no sensory deficit.

It is sometimes difficult on clinical grounds to distinguish between $C_8$, $T_1$ root lesions and ulnar nerve lesions. It can also be difficult to distinguish between ulnar nerve lesions at the elbow or wrist. Nerve conduction studies are often helpful in these circumstances.

# Question 5.14

There were no similar lesions found in the mouth of this patient.
1. What is the diagnosis?
2. At what level in the skin do these lesions occur?
3. What single investigation would help to confirm this diagnosis?
4. What is the prognosis?

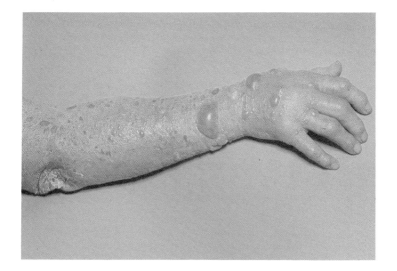

## Answer to question 5.14

1. Bullous pemphigoid.
2. The bullae are subepidermal.
3. A specific antibody for the basement membrane is found in the serum of most patients.
4. The prognosis is good with the lesions responding well to steroid therapy.

Bullous pemphigoid has to be distinguished from pemphigus vulgaris, erythema multiforme, drug eruptions and dermatitis herpetiformis. Bullous pemphigoid is usually found in elderly patients. In contrast to pemphigus vulgaris, the lesions are only occasionally found in the mouth. The blisters are deeper, tenser and less liable to rupture than those found in pemphigus vulgaris. A specific autoantibody to the basement membrane zone of the epidermis is found in 70% of patients. Pruritus may be a troublesome symptom but significant systemic disturbance is unusual. The prognosis is good with patients responding well to steroid therapy. Azathioprine is often used as well so that the dose of steroids may be kept to a minimum.

# Question 5.15

Of what condition is this blood film diagnostic?

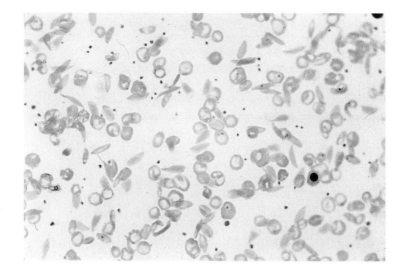

# Answer to question 5.15

Sickle cell disease.

The peripheral blood film shows gross poikilocytosis and the presence of multiple sickle cells. A few polychromatic erythrocytes and a normoblast are also present.

Sickling disorders consist of the heterozygous state for haemoglobin S (sickle cell trait) or the homozygous state (sickle cell disease). No haematological changes are seen in sickle cell trait and the diagnosis is confirmed by the finding of a positive sickling test (drop of blood mixed with 2% sodium metabisulphite) together with haemoglobins A and S on electrophoresis. Sickle cell disease is diagnosed by the finding of a variable degree of anaemia, elevated reticulocyte count, sickled erythrocytes on the peripheral blood film, positive sickling tests and a haemoglobin electrophoretic pattern characterised by the absence of haemoglobin A and the preponderance of haemoglobin S with a variable amount of haemoglobin F. Sickle cell trait should be present in both parents.

A similar clinical picture may result from the inheritance of the gene for some other abnormal haemoglobin, such as haemoglobin C, along with the Hb S gene.

# Question 5.16

What does this biopsy show?

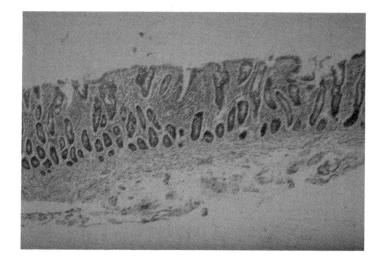

## Answer to question 5.16

Subtotal villous atrophy.

Although the typical features of coeliac disease are shown (villous atrophy, increased depths of the crypts and an inflammatory cell infiltrate) the degree of mucosal abnormality is better seen before fixation using a dissecting microscope. Other causes of these sorts of appearances include tropical sprue, kwashiorkor, hypogamma-globulinaemia especially if accompanied by *Giardia lamblia* infection, lymphoma, Whipple's disease and following radiotherapy.

In coeliac disease the mucosal abnormality lessens as one progresses down the intestine presumably related to the lesser exposure to gluten.

# Question 5.17

1. What two investigations should be performed?
2. What is the diagnosis?

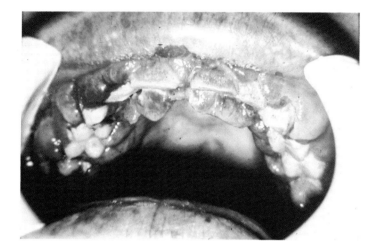

## Answer to question 5.17

1. Full blood count with film and a bone marrow.
2. Acute monocytic leukaemia.


Peripheral blood monocytes are widely accepted to be precursors of tissue macrophages in transit from the marrow. In acute monocytic leukaemia (M5 in the FAB classification of the acute non-lymphocytic leukaemias) monocytoid cells predominate. Monocytic leukaemias are found mainly in adult life. Most of the clinical features of acute leukaemia are shared by all types of the disease, and ulceration of the mucosa of the mouth with associated gingivitis is common. However gum hypertrophy is a particular feature of acute monocytic leukaemia.

# Question 5.18

What are the two differential diagnoses?

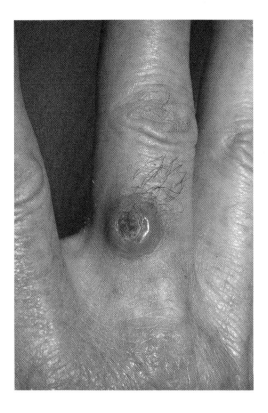

## Answer to question 5.18

Keratoacanthoma or squamous cell carcinoma.

Keratoacanthoma is a benign tumour thought to arise in the hair follicle. It should never reach more than 6 cm in diameter and is often mistaken for a squamous cell carcinoma. Usually these lesions resolve within 6 months but occasionally may take up to a year. It may be difficult to differentiate from a squamous cell carcinoma on histology. Treatment is usually conservative but excision may be necessary if their is doubt either clinically or histologically. They are more common in men than women and the patient often suggests that they are related to previous trauma. They are rare in people with racial skin pigmentation.

# Question 5.19

1. What is this condition?
2. What proportion of the patient's offspring will be similarly affected?

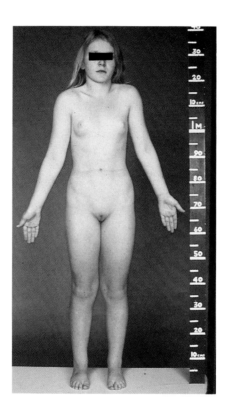

# Answer to question 5.19

1. Turner's syndrome.
2. None.


Turner's syndrome, or gonadal dysgenesis has a 45 XO karyotype. Patients usually present with primary amenorrhoea. Musculo-skeletal features include: a short stature with cubitus valgus, arched palate, short fourth metacarpal and shield chest. Osteoporosis, fused cervical vertebrae and abnormal carpus angles may be detected radiologically. Other abnormalities that may be seen include aortic coarctation, horseshoe kidney and lymphoedema. Streak gonads are usually present with infertility and poorly developed secondary secondary sexual characteristics. FSH elevation and chromatin negative 45 XO buccal smears confirm the diagnosis.

# Question 5.20

List 3 possible diagnoses of these scrotal lesions

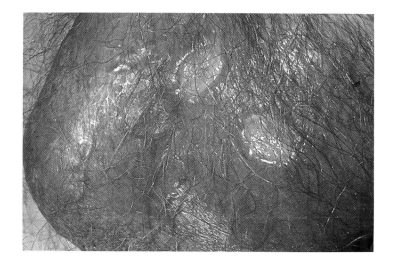

## Answer to question 5.20

1. Genital herpes
2. Syphilis
3. Chancroid
4. Donovanosis (granuloma inguinale)
5. Behçet's syndrome

The likelihood that a genital ulcer is due to a particular sexually transmitted agent varies from country to country. In the UK and USA genital herpes simplex is statistically most likely, followed by syphilis. In Africa chancroid is most common.

Herpetic vesicopustules are usually painful making the diagnosis easy if characteristic, but syphilis serology should always be performed since the two diseases may co-exist. Syphilitic ulcers are often painless and can be confirmed by dark ground illumination or serology using a rapid reagin test. If the lesion persists and serology for syphilis or chancroid is negative biopsy may be necessary to exclude Donovanosis (granuloma inguinale) or a carcinoma.

Non-infective causes include Behçet's syndrome with its triad of mouth ulcers, genital ulcers and ocular inflammation. Other causes of skin ulcers (e.g. pyoderma gangrenosa) rarely affect the genitalia.

# Bibliography

Fitzpatrick TB, Elsen AZ, Wolff K, Freedberg IM, Austen KF
(eds) 1979 Dermatology in general medicine, 2nd Edn.
McGraw-Hill, New York

Petersdorf RG, Adams RD, Braunwald E, Isselbacher KJ,
Martin JB, Wilson JD (eds) 1983 Harrison's Principles of
internal medicine, 10th Edn. McGraw-Hill, New York

Weatherall DJ, Ledingham JGG, Warrell DA (eds) 1983
Oxford Textbook of medicine. Oxford University Press

# Index